HEALTH for Life 1

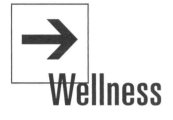 **Wellness**    **Relationships**   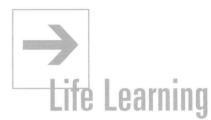 Life Learning

Author

Judith Campbell

Contributing Author
Wendy Mathieu

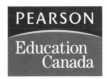
PEARSON

Education
Canada

Toronto

National Library of Canada Cataloguing in Publication

Campbell, Judith
    Health for life 1 / Judith Campbell; contributing author, Wendy Mathieu.

For use in grade 7.
ISBN 0-13-139892-X

1. Teenagers—Health and hygiene—Textbooks. I. Mathieu, Wendy
Lee II. Title. III. Title: Health for life one.

RA777.C328 2003 613'.0433   C2003-902938-7

ISBN 0-13-139892-X

Publisher: Susan Cox
Product Managers: Melanie Trevelyan, David Le Gallais
Managing Editor: Elynor Kagan
Senior Developmental Editor: Mary Kirley
Developmental Editor: Geraldine Kikuta
Production Editor: Milena Mazzolin
Copy Editors: Gail Copeland, Milena Mazzolin
Proofreading/Research: Gail Copeland, Susan Ginsberg, Dawn Hunter, Cara James
Production Coordinator: Zane Kaneps
Photo Research/Permissions: Amanda McCormick, Jeanne McKane
Art Direction and Design: Alex Li
Page Layout: Monica Kompter
Illustrators: Craig Terlson: pages 3, 21, 22, 30, 37, 46, 47, 77, 83, 89, 95, 101, 130, 134;
    Jane Whitney: pages 44, 45, 142–147
XML Coding: Louise Whitby
XML Production: Bhavin Desai
Cover Photograph: Corbis/Magma/Dann Tardif

1 2 3 4 5 TCP 08 07 06 05 04

Printed and bound in Canada

The publisher has taken every care to meet or exceed industry specifications for the
manufacturing of textbooks. The cover of this sewn book is a premium, polymer-
reinforced material designed to provide long life and withstand rugged use. Mylar
gloss lamination has been applied for further durability.

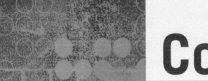

Contents

About This Book

Welcome to *Health for Life 1*— an exciting and fun way to explore some important topics about you and your health. Before you start to explore the information in this book, take a few minutes to read this section so that you will have a better idea of what *Health for Life 1* is all about.

Check out **In This Chapter** and **Key Terms** on the first page of each chapter to find out what topics you will be reading about and what key terms you will be learning. Each chapter also begins with a **Let's Go!** activity, which will get you thinking about the information you will explore in that chapter.

Look for **Over to You** activities, which are found throughout the chapters. These activities will give you a chance to be creative. You will have the opportunity to make a collage, work with other people, solve problems, come up with new ideas, draw cartoons, role-play scenes, and even do computer searches.

Certain Over to You activities are marked **Just for You.** These activities ask questions that are personal. You don't have to share your answers to these questions with other students. This information is especially for you!

Some activities have a blue portfolio icon beside them. This icon means you should save your work for this activity. You will be making a portfolio in Chapter 10 where you will keep this work. You will discover that a portfolio is a record of important information about who you are and the skills and talents that you have.

In each **Life Scene,** you will be reading about other students and some of their problems. In some Life Scenes, the students solve their own problems. In other Life Scenes, you will be asked to help the students find solutions.

Students have a lot of personal questions. You can read some of these questions and the answers in **Ask Sam.** You will also find interesting information in the margin. Be sure to read **Here's a Hint, Fast Fact,** and **VIP!** And check out the **Physical Activity Today** feature, which gives you a few quick and easy ways to add more activity to your day.

Enjoy yourself while you learn about *health for your life!*

Acknowledgements

My thanks to Dennis and Patrick Yandeau, two important teens who shared their wisdom and gave me insight throughout the writing of this book.

Thanks go also to the following reviewers:

Janaya Ellis, Ecole Rudolph Hennig School
Chris Gilbert, St. Andrew's Junior High School
Ralene Goldade, Calgary Catholic School District
Ross MacDonald, Lakeside Outreach School
Claire Macdonald, Senator Patrick Burns School
Peter Matsell, Memorial Elementary School
Barbara Milne, Edmonton Centre for Education
Lorrie Morales, Senator Riley School
Carol Scaini, Treeline Public School
Debbie Sprentz, Hamilton-Wentworth District School Board
YMCA Youth Substance Abuse Program

Medical Reviewer: Amish Parikh, MD, MEd, Faculty of Medicine, University of Toronto

Safety Procedures Reviewer: Peter Alexandrou, Canadian Red Cross

Judith Campbell

CHAPTER 1
Smart Learning

Key terms

unique, respect, learning style, personal learning style, self-talk, affirmation, visualization

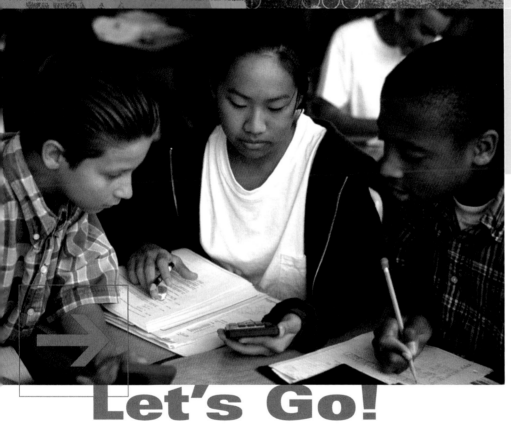

Let's Go!

→ In your notebook, list five reasons people go to school.

→ Share your list with a partner.

→ Together, combine the lists and rank the reasons, beginning with the most important.

Greetings! Here you are, right in front of this book, reading this page. Are you in a classroom, or at home doing your homework? Are you reading this book because it is part of your education? Whatever the reason, you are here—and you are learning.

In this chapter, you are going to learn about learning and the many ways that you can learn. You will consider some basics about school and learning and find some hints that will help you become a better learner.

Students: The Basics

Every class is made up of a group of students, each of whom has a combination of special interests, skills, talents, weaknesses, and strengths. Each student is a **unique** individual, including you.

unique: being the only one; unlike any other

You already know that some people do better than others in certain subjects. One person might do well in mathematics, but has to work hard to succeed in a physical education class. Another person might do well in art class, but struggles to write a good essay. People have strengths in different areas. That's true for you, too.

⌐ Over to You

Being unique has to do with combinations of personal traits. Think of at least three things that are special about you. Then list some ways you are similar to your friends. Create a collage or poem to show how a combination of your traits makes you a unique person.

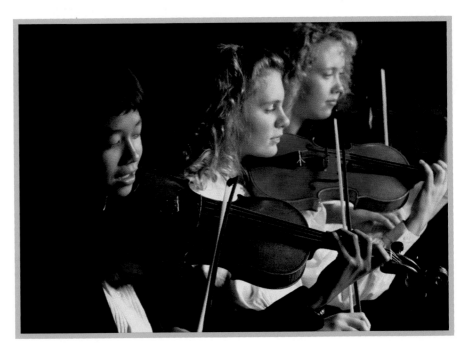

We are all alike in many ways, but we are also different. Everyone is unique.

New at School?

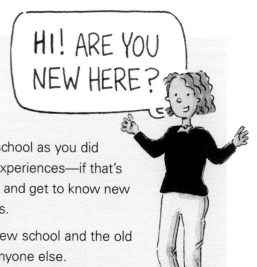

If you are new at a school, it might take some time and patience for you to feel like you fit in. Here are a few hints:

✳ Be open-minded. You won't feel as comfortable at your new school as you did at your old one. But if you dwell on your past friendships and experiences—if that's all you think about—you won't allow yourself a chance to meet and get to know new people. You might also miss out on your new school's activities.

✳ Don't make every conversation a comparison between your new school and the old one. These comparisons are more interesting to you than to anyone else.

✳ Make an effort to fit in. Don't wait for other people to approach you. Start by saying "hi" to the people around you.

✳ Remember: It takes time to get to know new people, and they need time to get to know you.

Teachers: The Basics

All teachers are trained to educate, explain ideas, and demonstrate skills, but not all teachers are the same. One teacher might joke a great deal, while another might be more serious. One teacher might want homework done one way, while another might have different expectations. One method of teaching is not necessarily better than another: it is just different. It is important to accept the differences and not want all teachers to be the same. Remember, too, that teachers are good people to talk to if you are having problems at school. They want you to be a successful student and they can give you help when you need it.

> ### Here's a Hint
>
> Be sure to learn how to do homework and assignments the way your teacher wants them done. Think about each of your teachers' expectations.

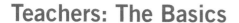
⤷ Over to You

1. Write your own definition of what a school is. List three ways that schools might differ from one another. In what ways should schools be the same?

2. Think about the best teacher you have had. What are five qualities that you liked about this teacher?

3. If you were teacher for a day, what qualities would make you a good teacher?

Classrooms: The Basics

All groups need rules or guidelines to function well. A class of students is no exception. Just as a sports team needs rules so that each member knows what is expected, so does a class.

Respect is the first rule of a classroom. It should be given to everyone, including the teacher. Students show respect for one another by accepting that there are many differences in the class. For example, you might understand a lesson before another student does. You respect that student when you allow him or her to ask questions, without any teasing or disruption from others.

Respect is essential in all class activities, including class discussions. Here are some basic rules for class discussions:

- Each person has the right to learn in school, and this right must be respected by each individual in the class.

- Each person has the right to speak or ask questions, without taunting, ridicule, or criticism.

- Each person has the right to pass, to choose not to speak. Some people prefer to contribute by actively listening. Listening is a way of showing respect for what is being said by others.

- Each person should use proper words and terminology in a discussion. Using appropriate language is part of showing respect.

respect: showing consideration for others

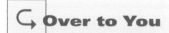
Over to You

Do you think that there are other important rules for class discussions? What are they?

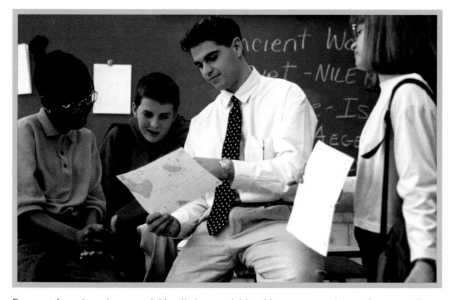

Respect for others is essential in all class activities. You respect others when you allow them to learn what you are learning.

Speak Up!

While everyone enjoys a moment of humour, continuous fooling around by a few individuals can be disruptive for the rest of the class. If you and your friends don't like this type of interruption, don't support the behaviour. Say something to the person or people involved. You might find that you get better results if you are polite.

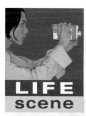

Consider each of the following classroom situations. What rules or guidelines can you suggest for each situation?

Emily

It's Social Studies, and the class is working on maps. Almost everybody is finding the assignment easy, but Emily feels completely lost. The teacher has explained the instructions twice, but Emily still doesn't understand what to do. The students who have finished are beginning to complain.

Ule

If a good laugh is what you want, Ule can provide it. Sometimes even the teacher smiles at Ule's jokes; other times, the teacher is annoyed because Ule uses up a lot of class time. One day the teacher didn't have time to remind the class about a test because Ule wasted time joking around. Some students forgot the test was the next day. That was definitely Ule's fault.

Iris

Iris is always late! Always! Last week she was late getting on the field trip bus, so the whole class was late for the museum tour. The tour guide had to rush through everything. And four students missed a special tour because the bus was so late that their tour was cancelled. Iris—the name means "always late."

Ted

Ted is just plain rude. He interrupts everybody and grumbles to himself. He curses quietly every time the teacher gives an assignment. When someone asks a question, Ted mutters something rude under his breath.

Harry

Extremely quiet—Harry never says anything. He never asks a question and he never answers a question. Harry has never said anything in any discussion, ever. Must say though, he's a pretty good student and OK to talk to out of class.

Get Ready for Success

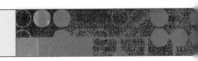

Now that you know the basics about school, you can start to think about how you can be successful. To be successful, you need to be prepared. How do you do this? A little organization can produce amazing results. Try the following ideas for better results at school and at home.

Get Organized for Better Results

At School

- Organize your notes in a binder or write them in a notebook.

- Bring your materials to class! This is so simple. You can't write without a pen. You can't read without your book. If you are prepared for class, you will feel more in charge of your learning.

- Pay attention in class. Take notes. Concentrate on what the teacher and other students are saying.

- Ask for an explanation as soon as you don't understand something.

- Use any free time you have at school to catch up on work that you might have missed and to get a start on the day's homework.

- Record due dates for assignments and dates for tests in a notebook or agenda. Always carry it!

- Have a "study buddy" who collects handouts and assignments for you when you are absent from school. And you can return the favour when this friend misses school. Exchange phone numbers or e-mail addresses so you can contact each other when necessary.

At Home

- Do your assigned homework. Homework contributes to increased learning.

- Work at a desk or table. Be sure your work area has a good light.

- Work in a quiet place. Music can be relaxing, if it is fairly quiet. Television is a distraction, and so is instant-messaging your friends.

- Have a study schedule and stick to it. Set aside an hour or so every school evening for homework and review.

- Spend a few minutes every night reading over your notes from the day's classes. If you wait until the night before a test, studying can seem like too large a task.

- Post a calendar over your study area and mark dates for assignments and tests.

- Take breaks when you study—maybe five minutes every half hour. And change subjects every once in a while to avoid boredom.

- Reward yourself when you have finished studying and completed your homework.

Learning Styles

A **learning style** is the way a person takes in information. Since people take in information in many ways, it is possible to have several different learning styles.

Like most people, you use different learning styles, but there are one or two styles that you probably prefer. The way you like to learn is your **personal learning style.** Your personal learning style could be the same style your friend uses. Or it could be different. No one style of learning is better than another: it is just different.

Learning by Seeing, Hearing, and Doing

How do you figure out what's cooking in a kitchen?

Do you read the menu?

Ask the cook?

Lift the lid of the pot and look?

Sniff the air, or taste a little bit?

We all use our senses—seeing, hearing, touching, smelling, and even tasting—to take in information. We all learn in slightly different ways, but there are three main ways we gather information—by seeing, by hearing, and by doing.

Here's a Hint

Always looking for something when you start your homework? Gather study supplies and store them in a plastic container or box. Your tool kit should contain pencils, pens, highlighters, an eraser, a sharpener, a self-stick notepad, a formatted disk, a dictionary, lined paper, scrap paper, tape, and small scissors.

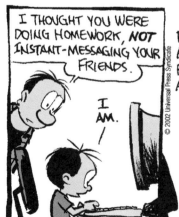
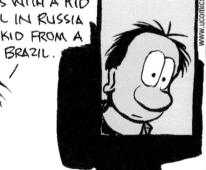
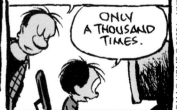

How have computers changed the way we take in information?

Learning by Seeing

Visual learners learn best by seeing what they are learning. They want to read and see pictures and diagrams.

Are you a visual learner? Do you:

- read words to understand something new?
- look at diagrams to figure out how things work?
- write notes in class to read and study later?
- prefer to read by yourself rather than have someone read to you?
- "see" a telephone number in your mind before you make a phone call?

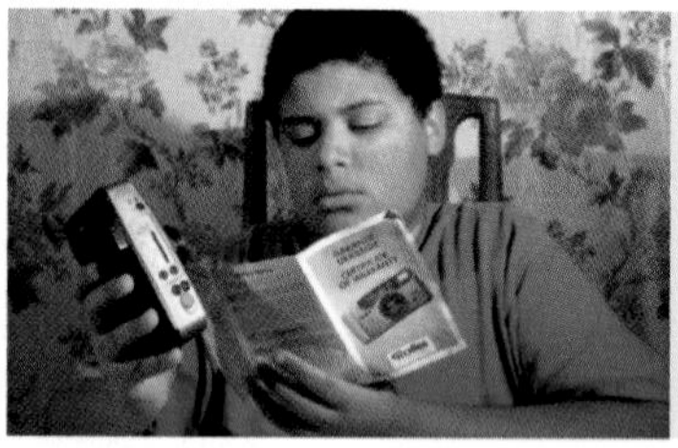

TIPS FOR BETTER VISUAL LEARNING

- Write notes when you are learning something new.
- Draw diagrams and pictures in your notes.
- Colour-code your notes using brightly coloured tabs and dividers.

Learning by Hearing

Auditory learners learn best by hearing and listening. They want to listen to new information and hear spoken explanations.

Are you an auditory learner? Do you:

- like to listen, even to yourself?
- learn more from what the teacher says than by reading?
- like class discussions and learn from them?
- prefer to tell a funny story in class rather than to write about it?
- "hear" a telephone number in your mind before you dial it?

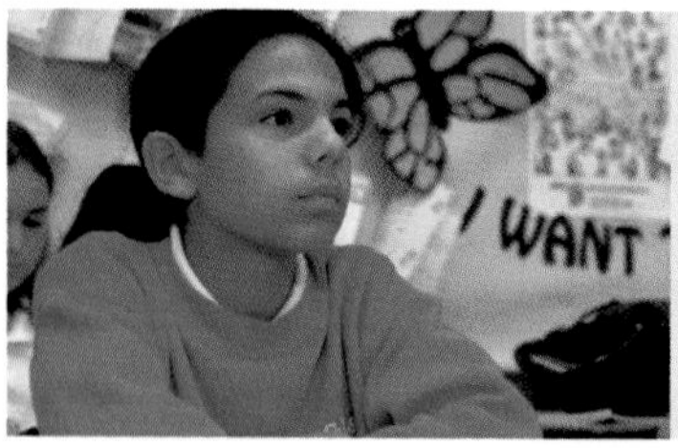

TIPS FOR BETTER AUDITORY LEARNING

- Listen carefully to what the teacher and others are saying.
- Read your notes out loud when you study, so you can hear the information.
- Participate in class discussions.

Learning by Doing

Kinesthetic learners learn best by touching and doing new things. They want a real physical connection to new information and like "hands-on" learning.

Are you a kinesthetic learner? Do you:

- learn best by "doing" instead of by reading or listening?

- want to try things before you get the instructions?

- use gestures and body language when you talk?

- want to be active when you are learning?

- punch in a telephone number without thinking and just let your fingers guide you?

TIPS FOR BETTER KINESTHETIC LEARNING

* Volunteer for role plays.

* Go to exhibitions and demonstrations; try the activity yourself.

* Use your finger to trace words that you want to remember.

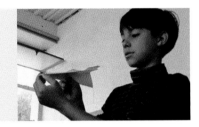

Learning Alone or Together

Do you prefer to learn alone, with friends, in a study group, or with the teacher? Your first answer might be "with friends." However, once you think about it, you might admit that, while you like having people around, you don't always get much done that way. How you prefer to learn often depends on what you are learning. For example, you might prefer to learn a subject such as math on your own. For other subjects, you might need a group discussion that allows you to share ideas with your classmates, ask questions out loud, and practise presentation skills. In other situations, you might need to ask a teacher about something you don't quite understand.

More Ways to Be Smart

Now you know that there are different learning styles and that you have a personal learning style. But do you know that you can also be smart in many ways? These "smarts" do not describe *who* you are. They describe the many ways you can be intelligent. If you know how to be smart in different ways, you can expand your ways of learning. Turn the page to find out about different kinds of smarts.

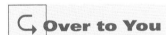 **Over to You**

Sometimes your personal learning style can let you down, and you just can't grasp new information. That's when you need to try something different. Review the different ways of learning mentioned in this chapter. Find two new ways of learning that you would like to try. Next time you have difficulty learning something, use these new ways of learning.

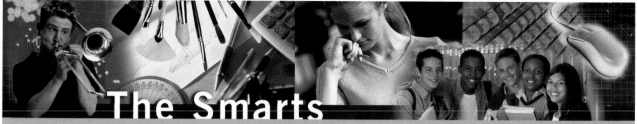

The Smarts

Word Smart

People with word smarts:

- use words well
- write well
- read often

They enjoy:

- reading books
- playing word games and solving puzzles
- having a good vocabulary
- writing for themselves

To expand **word smarts:**

- read a variety of books
- read aloud to others
- keep a journal

Picture Smart

People with picture smarts:

- create pictures in their mind to remember things
- understand maps, charts, and drawings

They enjoy:

- creating pictures and art
- drawing and doodling
- watching movies and videos

To expand **picture smarts:**

- imagine clear pictures of what you are learning
- illustrate stories with pictures and diagrams

Number Smart

People with number smarts:

- use numbers and logic
- organize things
- figure things out

They enjoy:

- working with numbers
- solving problems
- doing experiments

To expand **number smarts:**

- write outlines for studying
- do math; create your own questions

Music Smart

People with music smarts:

- hear music, melody, and rhythm in their environment
- connect music to other ideas
- create music

They enjoy:

- listening to music
- creating songs and lyrics
- playing instruments

To expand **music smarts:**

- sing, hum, play an instrument
- create your own songs and music

Body Smart

People with body smarts:	They enjoy:	To expand **body smarts:**
• move well and are coordinated • use their hands and fingers to do delicate work	• playing sports; doing gymnastics • dancing and acting • putting things together and taking them apart • working with their hands	• try doing something instead of just watching it be done • get involved in sports, gymnastics, dance, and acting

People Smart

People with people smarts:	They enjoy:	To expand **people smarts:**
• relate well to others • work well with others • are good leaders	• having good friendships • advising and helping people • being part of groups • being a leader	• be active in group discussions • be part of a team

Self Smart

People with self smarts:	They enjoy:	To expand **self smarts:**
• think about their own thoughts and feelings • work well on their own	• doing projects on their own • reading and reflecting	• take time to think about things • write thoughts in a journal

Nature Smart

People with nature smarts:	They enjoy:	To expand **nature smarts:**
• understand nature and natural things • observe patterns and connections in the environment	• being outside • observing nature • caring for pets	• enjoy time outside • create collections • learn about nature and animals

It is important for you to know your preferred style of learning so you can get better at using it. You can also learn how to learn in other ways. You don't have to be able to learn in all the ways you have read about here. You just need to know that all of these ways are possible. You get to choose the ways that work for you. It's not how smart you are, it's how you are smart.

Attitude? Positively!

How you think and feel influences how you learn. Wherever you go and whatever you do, you always bring your attitudes with you. No one makes an attitude for you. You create your own attitudes. Since it's your choice, you might as well think positively.

Positive attitudes open doors; negative attitudes close doors. So it is important to change negative attitudes into positive ones. Start by talking to someone who really matters—YOU.

Talk to Yourself

self-talk: a private talk that you have with yourself

Self-talk is the quiet talk that you have with yourself. It can be positive or negative. Positive self-talk gives you confidence and courage. Negative self-talk makes you believe you can't do something. The most effective thing you can do is change negative self-talk into positive self-talk.

For example, use positive self-talk before a pop quiz or test. Look at the test and say to yourself, "It's OK. Just be calm. Take two slow breaths. What do I know? What do I remember? I know the teacher talked about this yesterday." By the time you say your self-talk, the test will be underway, and you'll be ready to write the answers. You won't feel panicky.

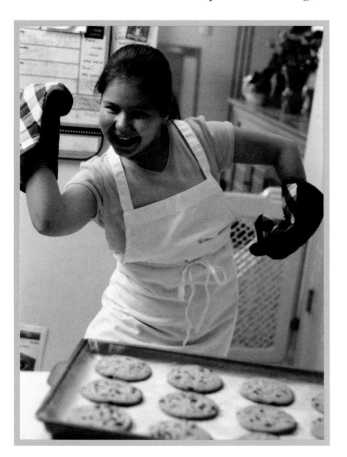

Self-talk and affirmations can give you confidence when you need it.

⤷ Over to You

Write three positive, encouraging statements that you can say to yourself before a class quiz. Now practise self-talk by quietly saying these statements over and over.

I Can Do That!

Another way to encourage yourself is to use **affirmations.** An affirmation is a strong, constructive statement about yourself. You might tell yourself, "I am a good listener" or "Everybody liked my class presentation." You say these statements to yourself any time you need to hear them. Affirmations can help you change your attitude from negative to positive, and they can make you believe more strongly in yourself. Many people, including athletes and performers, have affirmations they say to themselves at least once every day.

Affirmations can help you get past rough spots. When you are feeling down, like you can't succeed, an affirmation can bring you back and then set you on your way. That's how an affirmation helps you cope with obstacles. Use affirmations at these times: before you begin a project or test, when you are frustrated, when you need a reminder about how capable you are, any time!

Mental Movies

It is also important to *see* yourself doing something positive. How do you do this? Picture your success in your mind. A picture in your mind is called a **visualization.** You can create visualizations that work for you. Imagine what you want to have happen and play this scene over and over in your head, just like a movie.

affirmation: a positive statement about yourself

VIP! VERY IMPORTANT POINT

These 5Ws can change your attitude!
Answer these questions and change your attitude.
- What attitude do you have now?
- Why is this attitude hurting you or holding you back?
- What attitude do you need?
- What can you do to make this attitude part of you?
- When and where will you use this attitude?

visualization: a picture that you create in your mind

⌐ Over to You

1. Create two affirmations that you can use. For example, "I am a good student" and "I can write a successful test." Write down your affirmations. Now say each one. Will they work for you? Post these affirmations where you can see them, and read them often.

2. Create a cartoon that shows how an affirmation or a visualization can give someone a positive attitude.

◀◀ Now You Know

→ Each student has a unique combination of special interests, skills, talents, weaknesses, and strengths.

→ The first rule of a classroom involves respect for everyone, including the teacher.

→ There are different ways of learning. You have a personal learning style. You can learn using a combination of learning styles.

→ You can be smart in many different ways.

→ You create your own attitudes. You can choose to think positively. Positive self-talk and positive pictures of yourself in your mind can give you confidence.

↻ Over to You

1. Create an information booklet, brochure, or poster for people new to your school. Include the following details:

   • a map showing the location of the school in the community, bus stops, and other notable areas in the neighbourhood

   • a floor plan, showing the classrooms, gym, labs, and other significant rooms

   • information about the school, such as number of students and number of staff

   • reasons why your school is special

2. For one school week, track the number of hours you watch TV and spend at the computer. Then calculate the number of hours you spend at school in one week. Show your results on a table like the one below.

TV	Computer	School
Total hours:	Total hours:	Total hours:

a) What do these numbers tell you about how you spend your time?

b) Are there any changes that you would make? Explain.

3. In your notebook, make a table with the following headings:

Job	Useful Smarts
a movie stunt person	
a guide at an art gallery	
a disc jockey	
a journalist	
a hockey coach	
a florist	

a) Under the column Useful Smarts, list the different kinds of smarts each person would use on the job. Be creative in your thinking.

b) As a class, discuss the kinds of smarts needed for the different jobs.

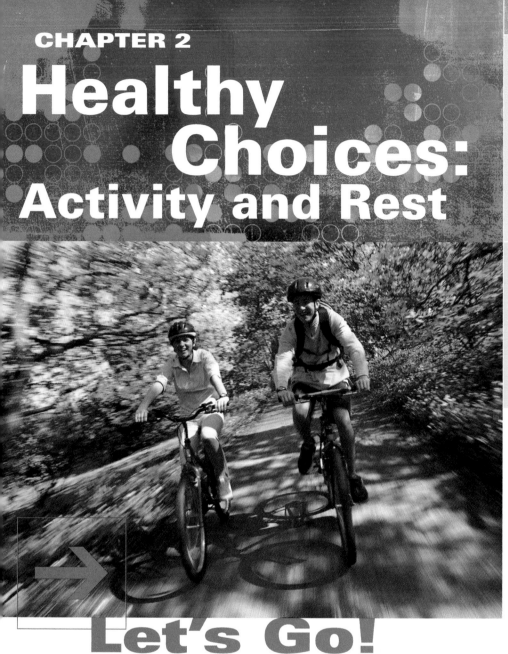

CHAPTER 2
Healthy Choices:
Activity and Rest

Key terms

standard,
personal standards,
goal,
sleep deprived,
REM sleep,
circadian rhythms

Let's Go!

→ Draw pictures, create a web, or write descriptions of five things you do to be healthy.

→ Write your own definition of what you think it means to be healthy.

You Are in Charge

Here's a Hint

To take care of yourself, you need to know as much as you can about your body and well-being. You use this information when you make choices and decisions about your health.

When you ask someone, "How are you?" you are recognizing that health is important. Being healthy is more than just not being sick. Health is one of the most important things you can have. Your health includes the physical, emotional, and social parts of you.

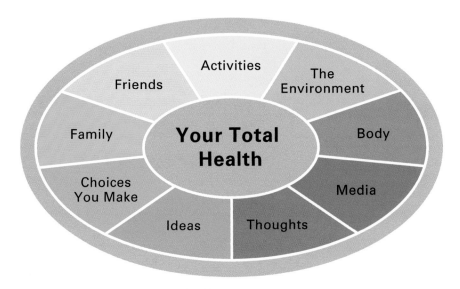

Everything around you affects your health.

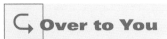

What are two choices you have made today that affect your health?

You are in charge of making choices about your health. You choose how much physical activity you get, how much sleep you get, and what you eat and drink. You will be making these choices throughout your life.

In this chapter, you will explore information that will help you make choices in two areas that affect your health: physical activity and sleep. You will also be gathering information about your personal health choices in these two areas, so recording this information in a journal or notebook is a good idea.

Standards and Guides for Your Health

standard: a level of achievement or activity that is required for something to be acceptable

A **standard** is a level that has to be reached or an amount that is needed for something to be acceptable. A standard sets a certain requirement. Your school has a certain standard that you have to meet in order to pass a test or move from one grade into another. Some standards indicate how we expect people to act in public. For example, knowing the standard of behaviour for eating in a restaurant will help you avoid embarrassment.

We all have **personal standards**—behaviours we expect from ourselves in different situations. Personal standards are helpful because they allow you to act without having to think out each step every time you act in a certain situation. For example, you know how to behave when you are in the responsible situation of looking after a young child.

There are also standards that can be applied to your health. These standards come from research and study. They are based on knowing what a human body needs to be healthy and remain at its peak. Standards are often explained in guides. Guides can be helpful when you are making choices about your health. *Canada's Physical Activity Guide for Youth* is an important guide that explains the standard of physical activity and shows how you can meet this standard.

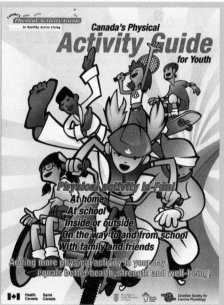

To get more information on physical activity, use a search engine to find *Canada's Physical Activity Guide for Youth* on-line.

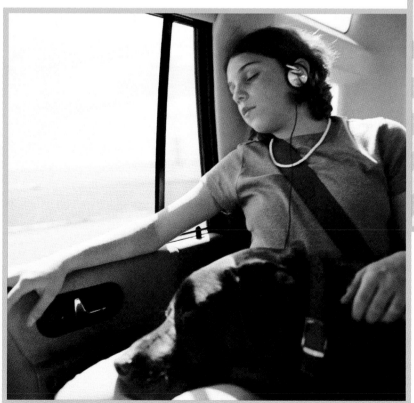

Safety standards can protect you from risk. Some of these standards become law. Seat belt laws protect people from injury.

Physical **Activity:**
What Your **Body** Needs

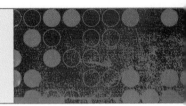

Stop Right Here!

- Before reading this section, you need to think back and make some notes.

- Think about the last 24 hours. What physical activities did you do?

- Make a chart in your notebook like the one opposite. List every physical activity that you did from this time yesterday until right now. For example, did you walk to school today? Did you have indoor soccer practice?

- Now estimate the number of minutes you spent doing each activity. For example, how long did it take you to walk home from the bus stop?

- With your chart, you are ready to read on.

24-Hour Physical Activity Chart		
Activity I Did	When	For How Long

Here's a Hint

Need some ideas to get you started? Try walking instead of getting a ride. Go skating, swimming, or bowling. Put on some music and dance.

Experts say that you need 60 minutes of physical activity every day. That's right—you need an hour of daily physical activity. Much of what you do each day involves physical activity. If you ride your bike to school, walk the dog, or shovel some snow, you have spent time being physically active just by doing ordinary activities. For some people, their daily physical activity also includes exercise, such as having a gym class, playing an outdoor game with friends, or swimming.

To figure out if you meet this standard, you need to know your current level of daily physical activity. You can measure activity time in 10-minute blocks. You need 6 blocks in your day to reach the standard of one hour of activity.

Increasing your daily physical activity is easier than you think. If you spend just a few more minutes each day doing the physical activities that you already do, and if you add some exercise to your day, you will be surprised to see how easy it is to get 60 minutes of activity into each day.

The Three Activity Groups

Health Canada identifies three types of activities that you need to do to keep your body healthy: endurance activities, flexibility activities, and strength activities.

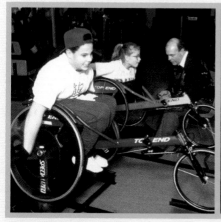 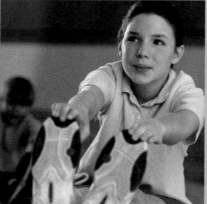 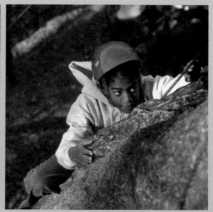

Endurance activities:
- make you breathe deeper
- make your heart beat faster
- give you more energy
- include wheeling (working a wheelchair), walking, rowing, cycling, swimming, skating, and dancing

Flexibility activities:
- involve bending, stretching, and reaching
- help you to move easily by keeping your joints mobile
- relax your muscles
- include yoga, Tai Chi, stretch exercises, raking the yard, and bowling

Strength activities:
- help to build your muscles
- help to keep your bones strong
- include everyday activities such as lifting and carrying groceries, climbing stairs, and wearing a backpack
- include exercises such as push-ups

↪ Over to You

- Take a look at your 24-Hour Physical Activity Chart (page 18). Add up the estimated time you spent doing each activity.

- Do you have 60 minutes of physical activity in your day?

- How do you think your activity choices and the amount of time you spent on them rate with the physical activity standard?

Not Yet	Almost Enough	Great Day!

Benefits of Physical Activity

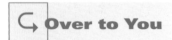

⟲ Over to You

As a class, brainstorm a list of all the physical activities you can think of. Which ones would you be willing to try?

Regular physical activity can eliminate that feeling of always being tired. It can improve circulation, which can help get rid of nagging little pains. Physical activity can also change that "who cares" attitude and do away with feelings of boredom.

Physical activity can improve your health. It can also help you:

✓ meet new friends

✓ maintain flexibility

✓ improve fitness

✓ feel good about yourself

✓ strengthen your heart

✓ sleep better

✓ build strong bones and strengthen muscles

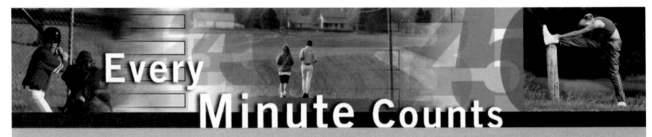

Every Minute Counts

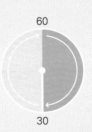

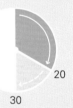

If you like to do vigorous activities that require more effort and energy, there's a bonus. You need to spend less time doing these activities to meet the daily standard for physical activity. Add up your activities in periods of at least 10 minutes each. Start slowly and build up.

You need **60 minutes** each day of light activity, such as:

- light walking
- volleyball
- stretching

You only need **30 to 60 minutes** each day of moderate activity, such as:

- brisk walking
- biking
- swimming
- dancing
- raking leaves

And you only need **20 to 30 minutes** each day of vigorous activity, such as:

- hockey
- basketball
- fast swimming
- fast dancing

You might favour one clock over another. Your choice of clock can also change each day.

Reach Your Goal by Making an Action Plan

Setting Your Goal

A **goal** is something you want to accomplish. Something you want to accomplish soon is a **short-term goal,** such as getting your homework done tonight before your favourite TV show.

Other goals can take more time and planning. These are **medium-term goals.** Reducing your TV watching by 30 minutes each day, or saving to buy a new computer game are medium-term goals.

Long-term goals are goals that might seem distant to you right now, such as planning what career you will choose.

Goals are personal, which means they belong to you. When you set a goal, think of the following things:

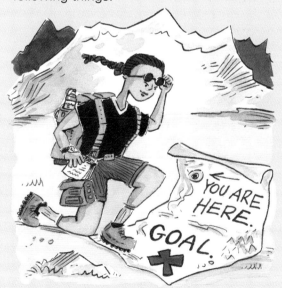

A goal takes you from where you are to where you want to be.

Goals   Your goal must be realistic. Don't set goals that are impossible to reach.

Obstacles   Recognize obstacles that might stop you from reaching your goal. Work out potential solutions.

Action plan   Prepare a step-by-step plan of how to reach your goal.

Look, listen, learn   You might need to do some research to find out what skills or information you need to achieve your goal.

Success   Measure successes along the way. Recognize when you have reached your goal. Feel good about your progress.

Making an Action Plan

Action plans allow you to move toward your goal one step at a time. To make an action plan, ask yourself these questions:

1. Where am I now?

2. Where do I want to be?

3. What actions or resources will get me there?

4. What is a realistic timeline for this plan?

5. How am I doing along the way?

6. How will I know if I am successful?

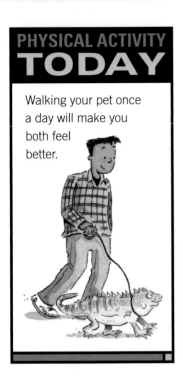

PHYSICAL ACTIVITY TODAY

Walking your pet once a day will make you both feel better.

⌐ Over to You

Now you do it. Set a goal to maintain or increase your level of physical activity each day. Make an action plan to reach this goal.

1. **Where am I now?** To find out, review the results from your 24-Hour Physical Activity Chart (page 18).

2. **Where do I want to be?** Do you need more activity each day? If so, how much more do you need: 10 minutes, 20 minutes, or more?

3. **What actions will get me there?** To decide, draw a weekly schedule based on the one below. Fill in your activities and plans for the week. Figure out when you have more time for physical activity. Add new activities where you think you could fit them in to your schedule.

	Monday	Tuesday	Wednesday
Before School	- walk to school	- computer chat	- walk dog
Morning		- gym class	

4. **What is a realistic timeline for this plan?** Can you start right away? Can you start after your music exam?

5. **How am I doing?** Check off each activity in your schedule once you have done it.

6. **How will I know if I am successful?** At the end of the week, measure your success. How did you do? Did you reach your goal?

Excuses! Excuses!

Making excuses is one of the most common ways to avoid doing something you don't feel like doing. Excuses are part of a negative attitude. They prevent you from reaching your goal. If you want to handle your excuses, you need to recognize them for what they are—just excuses. That's right. Sometimes our excuses are so good that we start to believe them. This does not make them good reasons for avoiding something we should do.

Think about all your excuses for not doing something physical. For example, maybe you don't want to go to soccer practice because you feel that you're not a very good soccer player. Now think about being positive and write a reason why each excuse is not enough to keep you from doing what you need to do.

Here's a Hint

Do some physical activity instead of thinking about what you can't do. The activity could be very simple: Put on your coat, go outside, walk around the block.

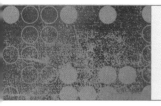

Sleep: What Your Body Needs

P hysical activity gets your body going, but you also need sleep to function properly. The amount of sleep people need varies from one individual to another. Some people need 10 hours of sleep to feel well rested; some need less than 6 hours. Teens need more sleep than children and adults do. Research shows that teens need between $8^1/_2$ and $9^1/_2$ hours of sleep each night.

Sleeping is a personal activity. Some people prefer to sleep in a cool room; some like it warm. Some people want the weight of heavy covers and blankets; some prefer a light sheet. Some people can only sleep in a room that is completely dark; others like some light.

Few teens get the amount of sleep their bodies need. Some even boast about how little sleep they get. The truth is that getting enough restful sleep is vital to good health. Sleep plays a large part in how you feel. Your choices about sleep affect how your body and mind work while you are awake. Your body needs sleep to perform well.

If you feel tired all the time, you might not be getting the sleep you need each night to restore your energy. You might be **sleep deprived.** Some teens try to make up for lost sleep on the weekends. This doesn't always work.

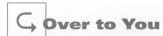

Fast Fact

You will spend almost one-third of your life sleeping.

⤷ Over to You

Describe the amount of light or darkness you need to sleep. What happens when you do not have the correct amount of light or darkness?

sleep deprived: not getting the amount of sleep each night that is needed to restore a sense of well-being and the feeling of being rested

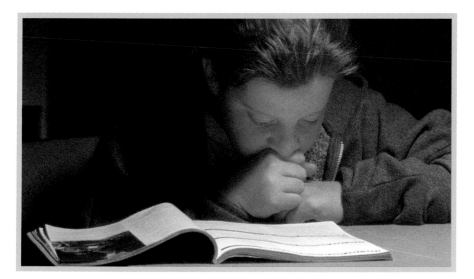

Many teens don't get the full amount of sleep their bodies need each night.

How People Sleep

Have you ever been so tired that you felt like you were asleep before your head hit the pillow? Actually, we fall asleep in stages. We start by drifting in and out of being awake and move to a stage where our heart rate and breathing slow down. Then we go into a deep sleep.

When we dream, we are experiencing **REM sleep** (rapid eye movement). Your eyes actually move rapidly under your eyelids during this phase of sleep. In a deep sleep, we switch from REM to non-REM sleep. Non-REM sleep is important because it is during this time that the body repairs and builds itself.

REM sleep: the stage of sleep when you dream

circadian rhythms: an internal "body clock" that causes people to feel sleepy or awake

Here's a Hint

Internal clocks do not change easily. If you are trying to change your sleeping pattern, you need to stick to your new timetable, even on weekends, for a month or more. It takes time for your circadian rhythms to reset.

So Why Are Teens So Tired?

Teens have special sleep needs. Why? Because there are major biological changes taking place in your body. And these changes affect your sleep. Everyone's sleep is determined by rhythms of the body called **circadian rhythms.** These rhythms work as the internal clock of the body. They tell us when to feel sleepy and when to wake up.

In teen bodies, the circadian rhythms are changing. Bodies that used to fall asleep early in the evening and wake up early in the morning might now find it difficult to fall asleep until much later at night. Teens who fall asleep late at night often have a difficult time getting up in the morning. This change in the internal clocks of teens is normal. In fact, it is necessary for the cycle of sleep to change as teens move to adulthood.

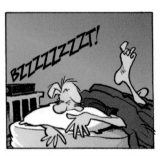
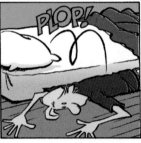
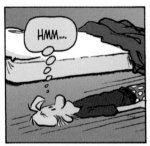
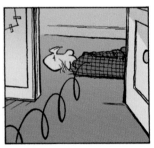
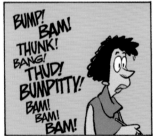
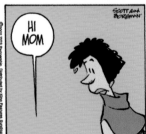
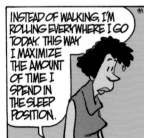
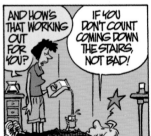

What are some other ways that Jeremy could get the sleep he needs?

What Lack of Sleep Can Do

Lack of sleep can have more serious consequences than simply making you cranky. When you don't get enough sleep:

- your body doesn't have enough time to do important repair work. You don't perform at your best.

- your immune system does not work as well. You are less able to fight off colds and other illnesses.

- your brain is less alert. You can't concentrate, especially on tests.

- your body is less coordinated. You are awkward, activities seem more difficult, and you are accident-prone.

When you get enough sleep, you just look better! Your eyes look brighter, your skin looks healthier, and you are more involved and interested.

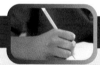

Ask Sam

Dear Sam,

Sometimes I just can't fall asleep at night, even though I'm really tired. I just lie in bed, thinking about things, especially the night before a test or something at school. Then I don't feel very well the next day. Like today. How can I fall asleep when I want to?

Tired and Growly

Dear Tired and Growly,

Everybody has problems falling asleep at times, so don't worry if it happens to you. The odd restless or sleepless night is normal. Don't fret about it. Fretting can keep you awake. Try imagining something boring and repetitive and see if this helps. If you still can't sleep, get up, find a comfortable place to sit, and read or listen to calming music for a while. When you begin to feel sleepy, try going back to bed. You'll be surprised how well this works.

Sam

Relaxation

You know that you need sleep, but do you know that you also need to relax? If you take some time to let your body and mind wind down for a little while, you can organize your thoughts, calm your body, relax your muscles, and enjoy the day. A few moments of relaxation can give you energy for the rest of the day.

How do you like to relax when you are on your own? How do you relax when you are with family or friends? Which form of relaxation works best for you?

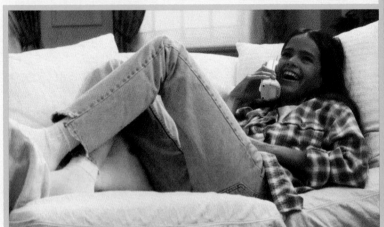
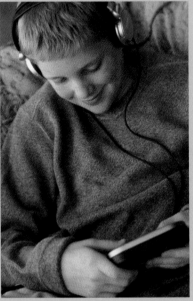

Relaxing means spending time doing something you enjoy. You might like listening to music, talking to friends, reading, or just spending some quiet time alone.

↳ Over to You

1. a) For one week, record the time you go to bed each night and the time you get up. Add up the total hours of sleep you had for the week. If a teen needs $8\frac{1}{2}$ hours of sleep a night, calculate the hours of sleep a teen should get for a one-week period. How does this figure compare with your total amount of sleep for the week?

   b) If you need more sleep, set a personal goal to get more sleep for one week. Start by reviewing the action plan questions on page 21. Then create your action plan for one week. Write down what you can do each evening to get to bed earlier. Post your plan somewhere in your bedroom where you can see it each night.

2. Create a cartoon that shows why relaxation is important to health.

◀◀ Now You Know

→ You are in charge of making healthy choices about your physical activity and sleep.

→ A standard is a level that has to be reached or an amount that is needed for something to be acceptable. There are standards that can be applied to health.

→ We have personal standards—behaviours we expect from ourselves in different situations.

→ Goals are achievements we want to fulfill. They can be short term, medium term, or long term.

→ Action plans help you achieve your goals.

→ Excuses can keep you from doing what you really want to do.

→ Teens need more sleep than children and adults do. Getting enough sleep is vital to good health.

→ Teens experience major biological changes that affect their sleeping patterns.

↻ Over to You

1. a) Survey three students in your class. Ask them the following questions. Record their answers.

i) Approximately how many minutes of physical activity did you do yesterday?

ii) How does your activity level compare with the standards in *Canada's Physical Activity Guide for Youth*?

iii) What new activities would you like to try?

b) Present your findings to the class in a visual way. It could be a graph, collage, drawing, or poster.

2. Create a saying or design a bumper sticker that would encourage people to be physically active.

3. Make a list of two strength activities, two endurance activities, and two flexibility activities that you can do outdoors. Make a similar list of activities that you can do indoors. Next time you need a new activity, try one of these.

4. We have all made excuses for not doing something we don't feel like doing. List as many excuses as you can for not doing some physical activity. With a partner, discuss your list and suggest ways to deal with each excuse.

Key terms

nutrients,
*Canada's Food Guide
to Healthy Eating*,
food groups

CHAPTER 3
Healthy Choices:
Food for Thought

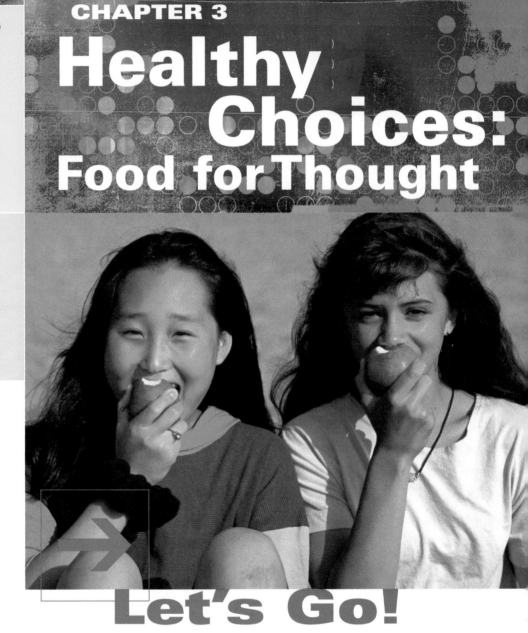

Let's Go!

→ Do you ever eat junk (less healthy) food?

→ How can you encourage yourself to make healthy food choices?

Food: What You **Need**

I n the last chapter, you learned how to set goals and create action plans for physical activities and amount of sleep. In this chapter, you will set goals and create an action plan for healthy eating. You will also design your own food guide.

Canada's Food Guide to Healthy Eating

Your body needs nutritious foods to keep it running. Nutritious foods are foods that contain **nutrients,** substances your body needs but cannot make on its own.

It would be difficult to choose foods quickly if you had to stop and think about the nutrients in everything you ate. *Canada's Food Guide to Healthy Eating* does the work for you. The Guide outlines groups of healthy foods. It also provides instructions for how to choose the foods you require each day from each group in order to get the nutrients you need. The instructions are simple and easy to learn. The different groups are known as **food groups.**

Every day a teen body needs:

- 5–12 servings of grain products

- 5–10 servings of vegetables and fruit

- 3–4 servings of milk products

- 2–3 servings of meat and alternatives to meat

Examine the table on the next page to make your food choices easier.

nutrients: substances your body cannot make but does need in order to work properly

food groups: foods with similar nutrients

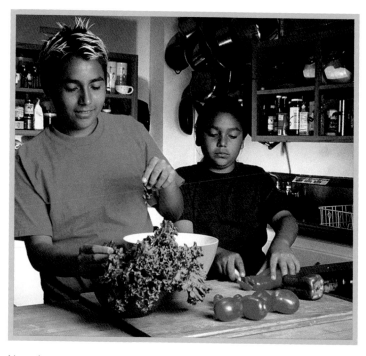

Next time you need a snack, try a salad, fresh vegetables, or fruit.

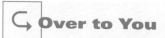
Over to You

To get more information on healthy eating, use a search engine to find *Canada's Food Guide to Healthy Eating* on-line.

Food Choices

Food Group	Some of the Foods in Group	Examples of Single Servings
Grain Products 5–12 servings per day	breads, bagels, pitas, biscuits, crackers, cereal, rice, all noodles and pastas	- 1 slice of bread - 1 cup (250 mL) of cold cereal - 1/2 cup of pasta or rice
Vegetables and Fruit 5–10 servings per day	carrots, broccoli, potatoes, apples, bananas, juice, raisins, and any other vegetable or fruit you can think of	- 1 medium-sized vegetable or fruit - 1/2 cup of juice - 1 cup of salad - 1/2 cup of fresh, frozen, or canned vegetables or fruit
Milk Products 3–4 servings per day (for youth, 10–16 years)	milk, cheese, yogourt, ice cream	- 3/4 cup of yogourt - 1 cup of milk - 2 slices (50 g) of cheese
Meat and Alternatives 2–3 servings per day	meat, poultry, fish, beans, eggs, peanut butter, tofu	- 50–100 g of meat, poultry, or fish - 125–250 mL of beans - 1/3 cup of tofu - 2 tablespoons of peanut butter

What Size Is a Serving?

Canada's Food Guide to Healthy Eating recommends a certain number of servings from each food group every day. It gives a range of servings because bodies come in different sizes and have different needs. But how much is a serving? One way to estimate servings is to use the handy guide below.

Handy Serving Sizer

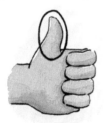

A thumb equals 25 g of most cheeses, so two thumbs equals one serving of cheese.

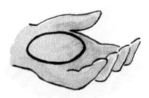

A palm equals one serving of meat, fish, or poultry. That's without fingers and thumb!

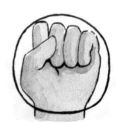

A fist equals one cup, so a fist size of salad would be one serving of vegetables. And a fist size of pasta or rice would be two servings of grains.

Other Ways to Estimate Servings

Hands come in different sizes, so you may need other ways to help you estimate the size of a serving. You can use everyday objects as a guide to how many servings you are eating. The chart below shows the approximate size of one serving.

What Does One Serving Look Like?

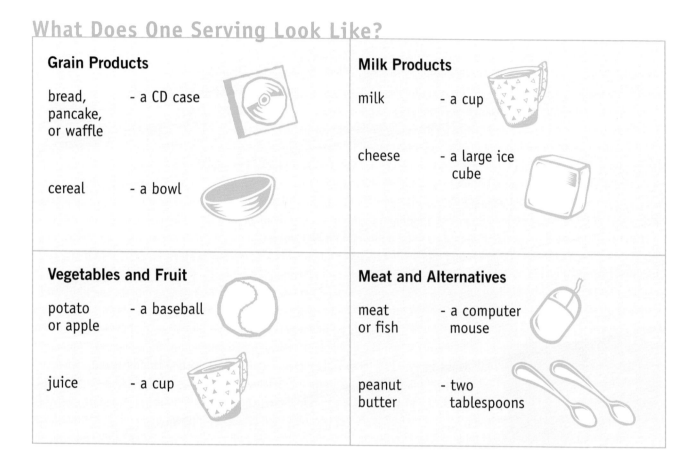

Grain Products

| bread, pancake, or waffle | - a CD case |
| cereal | - a bowl |

Milk Products

| milk | - a cup |
| cheese | - a large ice cube |

Vegetables and Fruit

| potato or apple | - a baseball |
| juice | - a cup |

Meat and Alternatives

| meat or fish | - a computer mouse |
| peanut butter | - two tablespoons |

Combination Foods

A casserole, stew, and stir-fry are all examples of **combination foods** because they contain a variety of different foods. To figure out the number of servings from each food group that you have eaten in any combination food, do the following:

- List the main foods in the dish. For example, a stir-fry might be made up of rice, vegetables, and meat.

- Now estimate how much you ate of the main foods in the dish. Did you eat the size of a baseball, a computer mouse, or your thumb?

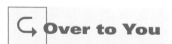 **Over to You**

Pizza is a combination food. Think about your favourite pizza. Then estimate the amount of diffent foods you eat when you have a slice.

Start Now!

- For one whole day—24 hours—write down everything you eat and drink.
- Record this information in a table like the one below.
- Keep your table handy so that you don't forget to record any items.
- Estimate how much of each food you eat during this time. You will have to make a smart guess about some foods. Look at the food before you eat it and estimate the amount.
- Don't forget to record how much water you drink.
- You will need this information at the end of the chapter.

24-Hour Food Log

When	What I Ate and Drank
6:00 a.m.	
8:00 a.m.	
10:00 a.m.	

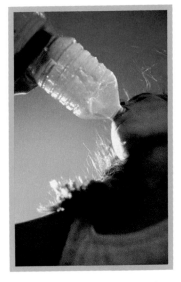

Drinking a lot of water every day is important. Water regulates your body temperature so that your body can function properly.

A Note on Water

Making healthy food choices is not just about what you eat. Water is vital to your body as well. Your body is a large collection of cells, and every cell needs water. Water transports nutrients to the cells. It also transports waste products out of your body. Soft drinks and coffee are not a substitute for water. They often contain caffeine and other ingredients.

↪ Over to You

1. Do the following in your notebook:

   a) Write down your favourite fruits and vegetables.

   b) List three fruits and vegetables you eat when you are at home.

   c) Now list three fruits and vegetables you choose when you eat out.

2. Make the same kind of list for your favourite grain products, milk products, and meat or alternatives to meat. Keep these lists. You'll be using them later in the chapter.

Vegetarian?

Some people choose not to eat meat at all. For some, eating meat goes against their religious beliefs; others don't eat meat because they are concerned about animal rights or the environment. For some people, meat may be too expensive, while others might feel that it is unhealthy to eat meat.

Meat contains many important nutrients, including protein and iron. People who don't eat meat or those who only eat small amounts of meat, need to get these nutrients from other foods.

Protein is found in a wide variety of foods, including nuts, peanut butter, lentils, tofu, soy milk, cereals, breads, and vegetables. Foods with iron include chickpeas, lentils, baked beans, spinach, and dried fruit.

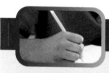

Ask Sam

Dear Sam,

My friend has decided to become a vegetarian. He eats a lot of vegetables, cheese, and different grains. But sometimes he also eats chicken. He said it's OK if a vegetarian eats chicken. Is he really a vegetarian?

Curious

Dear Curious,

There are different ways to be vegetarian. Not all vegetarians avoid the same foods. Some vegetarians eat poultry, fish, eggs, and dairy foods, but no meat or other animal products. Some vegetarians eat dairy foods and eggs, but no poultry, fish, meat, or other animal products.

A vegan is a person who only eats food from plant sources, no animal foods of any type.

Whichever kind of vegetarian your friend is, he should remember to include foods that provide the nutrients he would otherwise get from meat.

Sam

A Personal Food Guide

Canada's Food Guide to Healthy Eating gives general guidelines for healthy eating. The guidelines are based on five main principles:

* Enjoy a variety of foods.
* Emphasize cereals, breads, other grain products, vegetables, and fruit.
* Choose lower fat dairy products, leaner meats, and food prepared with little or no fat.
* Achieve and maintain a healthy body weight by enjoying regular physical activity and healthy eating.
* Limit your intake of salt and caffeine.

Canada's Food Guide allows you to make many food choices while you follow its principles. Using these principles, you can make your own personal food guide to healthy eating. You will be able to use your personal food guide when you are in a real hurry. Just look at your guide and choose the foods you like from each food group. Voila! A healthy meal. Or let's say you are really hungry and need something to eat right now. Take a quick look at your guide and pick out the foods on your list that are quick to get. This will help you eat healthy foods *and* foods you like. With your own personal food guide, you will be in charge of the foods you eat. And you will be making healthy choices.

Once you have made your personal food guide, you might want to post it on the fridge so you can see it when you need it. On the next page, you'll find an example of one student's personal food guide.

The student we will be looking at is Dennis. Dennis is an active student at school. He likes to get involved in school activities and hangs out with his friends when he can, like during lunchtime. Outside of school, Dennis spends most of his time at gymnastics practice. He often eats in the car as his mom or dad drives him from school to gymnastics lessons. On Saturdays, Dennis takes a lunch to the gym. He says he is hungry most of the time!

Here's a Hint

When you make your food guide, include a variety of foods from each food group. If you have only a few choices, you will quickly grow bored with your selection. You will get tired of eating the same few items over and over.

Dennis' Personal Food Guide

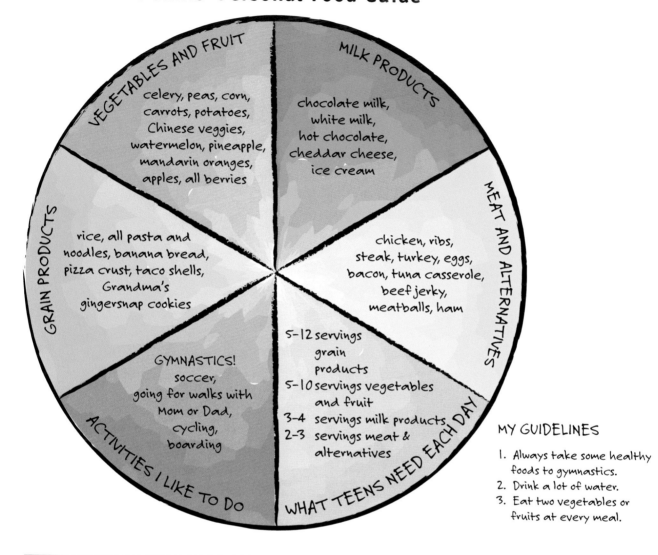

VEGETABLES AND FRUIT
celery, peas, corn, carrots, potatoes, Chinese veggies, watermelon, pineapple, mandarin oranges, apples, all berries

MILK PRODUCTS
chocolate milk, white milk, hot chocolate, cheddar cheese, ice cream

GRAIN PRODUCTS
rice, all pasta and noodles, banana bread, pizza crust, taco shells, Grandma's gingersnap cookies

MEAT AND ALTERNATIVES
chicken, ribs, steak, turkey, eggs, bacon, tuna casserole, beef jerky, meatballs, ham

ACTIVITIES I LIKE TO DO
GYMNASTICS! soccer, going for walks with Mom or Dad, cycling, boarding

WHAT TEENS NEED EACH DAY
5–12 servings grain products
5–10 servings vegetables and fruit
3–4 servings milk products
2–3 servings meat & alternatives

MY GUIDELINES
1. Always take some healthy foods to gymnastics.
2. Drink a lot of water.
3. Eat two vegetables or fruits at every meal.

↪ Over to You

1. It's time to create your own food guide to healthy eating.

a) Start by reviewing the list of your favourite foods from each food group (page 32). Include these foods in your guide and add as many new foods as possible.

b) Now write three rules that will remind you how to eat healthy. Make these simple so you can remember them.

c) Healthy food choices should be combined with physical activity, so create a list of physical activities that you enjoy.

d) Create a design for your guide. You could use colour, graphics, and other elements that appeal to you.

Influences on Food Choices

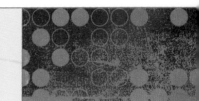

Do you always choose to eat healthy foods? Many people answer "Not all the time. I try but I don't always do it." Why don't people always choose healthy food? Why do some people eat more than they need to eat, while others eat less? The answer is because many things influence food choices.

Some people do not know which foods keep a body healthy. Others might not know the right amount of food to eat. You now know these things. So what influences you? Here are some ideas:

Personal food preferences: You eat the foods you like. You choose foods that taste good to you. You also make choices based on what you think is good for you.

Influence of friends and peers: When you are with friends, you might choose to eat the same foods they eat, or similar foods. Friends and peers do not force one another to eat certain foods, but many times, teens eat alike. As an example, just think about a group of friends eating at a fast-food place. Your choices can be influenced by what other people like to eat.

Money to spend: When you eat out, you choose the foods that you can afford. At a store, restaurant, or fast-food place, you can choose only what you can pay for.

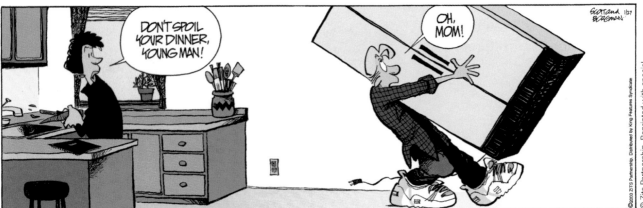

Influence of family: When you are at home, you eat what your family buys and eats. Chances are, some of your favourite foods are ones that your family eats. Do you have a favourite meal or birthday cake? Home is also where you learn family traditions about food.

Hunger: When you are hungry, you eat what you can find quickly and prepare easily.

Available time: When you are in a hurry, you eat food that is available to you and that won't take much time for you to prepare. Perhaps you grab a sandwich, a piece of fruit, or you buy fast food. Not having enough time influences your choice of what to eat.

Influence of advertising: The world of food is filled with advertising that tries to convince you to choose one food over another without thinking about whether it is good for you. Advertising is everywhere—on television, on billboards, in newspapers, even on food wrappings and boxes.

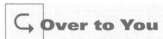
Over to You

Draw a diagram like the one below, with *you* in the middle. In each circle, write one influence and give an example of how that influence affects your food choices. For example:

Hunger: I'm really hungry after school so I snack a lot.

Factors That Influence Your Food Choices

- Available Time
- Influence of Advertising
- Hunger
- Influence of Friends and Peers
- Money to Spend
- Personal Food Preferences
- Influence of Family

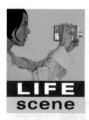

Food for Thought

Now you are ready to read about four teens who talk about problems they had with choosing healthy food. As you read their stories, think about how their food choices were influenced. Then think about what they did to solve their problems.

Hamed

I am STARVING when I get home from school. The first thing I do is check out the fridge, then all the cupboards. I eat pretty much anything I can find that doesn't take time to prepare. That means a lot of cookies, chips, and pop.

Hamed's solution

I figured out that I need two lunches—one for school and one for after school. Now I make myself two lunches, all out of foods I like. And I stay away from too much junk food. I take one lunch to school and leave the other one in the fridge. When I come home, I open the fridge and there it is—my own perfect after-school snack!

Carmen

I am sort of on a diet. Some days I don't eat anything for as long as I can stand it. Yesterday I didn't have anything all day except some gum, but then I blew it. After school I had large fries, a pop, and half my friend's giant cinnamon bun. When my mom made me have some dinner, I felt sick.

Carmen's solution

Hi. This is Elle, Carmen's friend. Listen, Carmen knows about eating healthy, but she was fooling herself on this weird diet. But the other day, a guy teased her about eating "garbage," so she decided to make some changes. Now she has something to eat before school: strawberry yogourt and raisins. She also carries two fruit chew bars in case she gets hungry during the day. Sometimes she even takes a lunch to school.

Mae

Everybody in our house is so busy that we eat out almost every night. I don't mind because I get to choose my own dinner. Chicken, burgers, shrimp, tacos, pizza, and falafels are just a few choices. At school I learned about *Canada's Food Guide to Healthy Eating*, and I wondered how this guide could fit in with my eating habits.

Mae's solution

This problem was pretty easy to solve. I spent a few minutes seriously looking at the Food Guide. Now I make sure to order a salad, or veggies, and milk with each meal. I also try to avoid fried foods as much as possible. Every once in a while, I recheck the Food Guide just to make sure I'm on track.

Miles

I choose cereals based on how cool the commercial is on TV, and what toys or gimmicks are inside. At the coffee shop, I order the special that is advertised on the chalkboard by the door. It doesn't matter what it is. A lot of sugar can make anything taste good.

Miles' solution

After learning about nutrition in Health class, I decided to try to eat healthier. I started reading cereal boxes to see what nutrients were in which cereals. Now I eat only the healthy cereals. At the coffee shop, I order anything that has mostly milk in it. I tell people it's what makes me big and strong!

⤷ **Over to You**

1. Using the diagram on page 37, identify the factors that influenced the choices made by each of the teens in Life Scene.

2. Write a scenario like the ones in Life Scene. In your scenario, show how friends can be a positive influence on food choices.

3. Choose two of the teens in Life Scene who could use more information about choosing healthy foods. What are two suggestions you could give each of them for making better food choices?

◀◀ Now You Know

→ *Canada's Food Guide to Healthy Eating* makes choosing healthy foods easier by putting foods into four basic food groups.

→ The four food groups are grain products, vegetables and fruit, milk products, and meat and alternatives.

→ There are many ways to estimate a food serving.

→ Creating your own food guide can help you make better food choices.

→ To be healthy, you need a combination of physical activity and healthy foods.

→ Your food choices are influenced by many factors. These include family, friends and peers, advertising, available time, hunger, money, and personal preferences.

↺ Over to You

1. In the last chapter, you set goals for increasing physical activity and getting more sleep. Now you can do the same for making better food choices. Once you have set your goal, make an action plan to help you reach it. Make your plan for one week.

   a) Begin by reviewing your 24-Hour Food Log. Compare your food log with *Canada's Food Guide to Healthy Eating* and the personal food guide you made on page 35. How did the food choices from your food log compare with both guides?

   b) Using this information, set a goal. Maybe your food log shows that you haven't been eating enough vegetables. Maybe it shows you have been skipping breakfast. Your goal would be to solve these problems.

   c) Create an action plan that will help you make better choices every day. Discuss this plan with your family. How can this plan work at home? How can this plan work when you eat away from home?

   d) After you have tried your plan for a week, you can decide if you were successful. Did you reach your goal? How do you know? Write a summary explaining how the plan worked. Is there anything else you would change? 📁

Body and Mind

Key terms

puberty, hormone, growth spurt, personal reflection, consumer, target group, media, body image, healthy body image

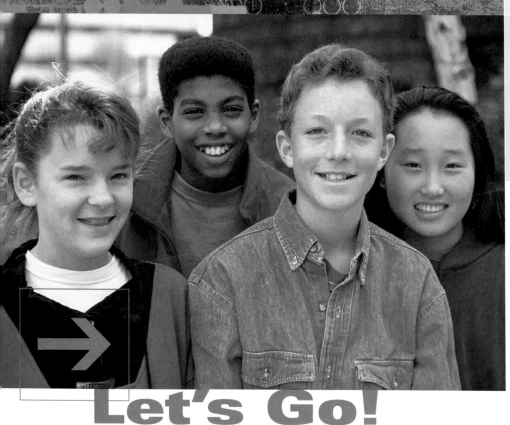

Let's Go!

→ In your journal, name two adults you could talk to about personal matters. These are two people you trust and feel comfortable with. This may take some serious thinking on your part, but it is important to have these names in the back of your mind in case you need them sometime. This is personal information.

Changes, Changes

A s a teen, you will be facing many changes. Some of these changes will be physical. Some will be related to new choices you need to make. In this chapter, you will learn about some of these changes and choices. You will also discover ways to create healthy images of yourself as you go through changes.

Hello, Puberty!

puberty: a stage of development between childhood and adulthood when a person matures

Puberty is the process that changes you from a child to a young adult. Puberty begins before your teen years and lasts until your late teens or later. Even if your body has not changed much yet on the outside, you are in puberty. You will be experiencing a lot of changes over the next few years. Puberty is an exciting process, and it will change you forever!

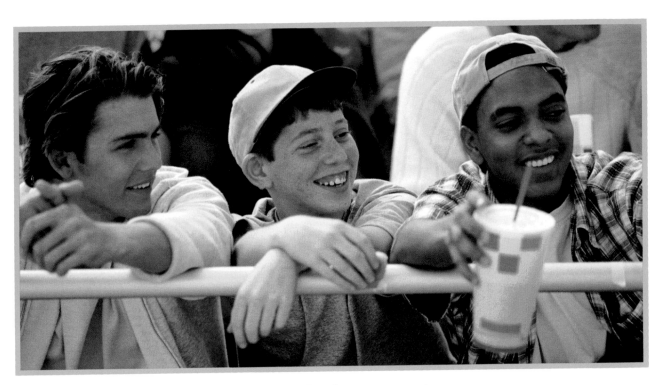

During puberty you experience changes you can see, as well as changes you cannot see.

Puberty Is Personal

How and when puberty happens to you is personal. The start time and the length of puberty is different for each body. Your puberty will start and end on its own timetable.

You cannot control or change the rate that your body goes through puberty. However, this is your chance to learn about puberty so that you will understand the changes as they happen.

As you go through puberty, there will be many changes in how you look, feel, act, and think. You cannot see all of these changes, so you cannot judge where you are in the process of puberty. Your body may seem ahead of others in physical changes, or you may worry that your body will never change. It is important to remind yourself of the following points:

- There are many changes that cannot be seen, and you can be changing in these ways without looking different.

- Each person has a personal puberty timetable.

- Each person reacts differently to the changes that are taking place.

With all of this happening, it is no wonder each teen experiences puberty in a personal way.

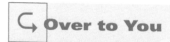

Over to You

Find an old photo of yourself. In what ways do you look different? In what ways do you look the same?

The Puberty Process

The process of puberty begins in the brain with hormones. A **hormone** is a substance produced in one area of the body and then transported through the bloodstream to another area of the body, where it causes change or growth.

Many different hormones play a role in puberty. Some hormones cause changes in every teen's body. Changes begin as your body starts to produce hormones that cause bones and muscles to grow. There are specific hormones that cause changes only in the female body. There are other hormones that cause changes only in the male body. Some of the same changes happen to both females and males. Some changes are visible; some are not. Changes during puberty take place over several years. By the time your body has gone through all the changes, you will have developed into a young adult.

hormone: a substance produced by the body that causes some changes or growth

Puberty and Body Changes

There are many physical changes that happen during puberty that you can see. Here are just a few of them.

Skin

A change in your skin may be one of the first things you notice. Your skin has oil glands, especially on your face, neck, shoulders, chest, and back. Your skin may feel oily as these glands become active and release oil through openings called pores. Some pores could become blocked with oil, causing the following:

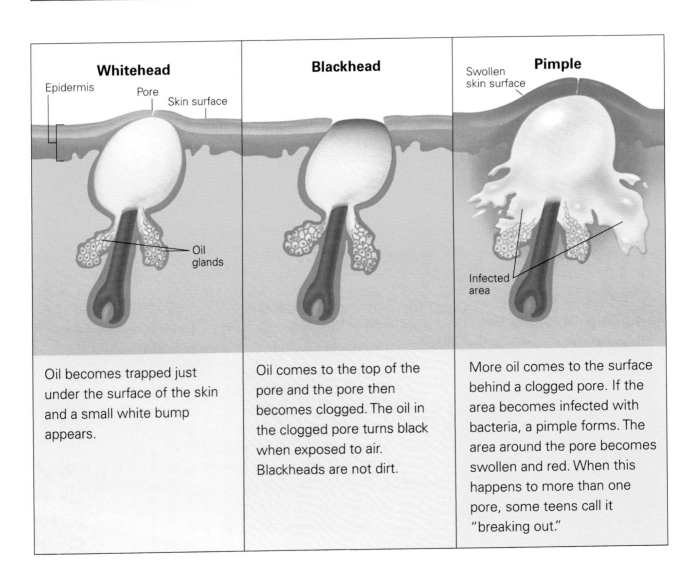

Whitehead

Epidermis   Pore   Skin surface

Oil glands

Oil becomes trapped just under the surface of the skin and a small white bump appears.

Blackhead

Oil comes to the top of the pore and the pore then becomes clogged. The oil in the clogged pore turns black when exposed to air. Blackheads are not dirt.

Pimple

Swollen skin surface

Infected area

More oil comes to the surface behind a clogged pore. If the area becomes infected with bacteria, a pimple forms. The area around the pore becomes swollen and red. When this happens to more than one pore, some teens call it "breaking out."

Sweat Glands

Body odour happens now because your sweat glands are starting to work. Now there is more sweat, or perspiration as it is more delicately named, under your arms and on your feet, just to mention a couple of places. Everybody gets his or her own particular body odour. Other people might notice your body odour before you do.

Hair

With puberty comes hair growth in many areas of your body, including legs and underarms. Over time, this hair becomes thicker and darker. Later in puberty, boys grow facial hair.

Voice

During puberty, your voice changes and becomes deeper. This happens to both girls and boys, but it is more obvious in boys because there is a bigger change in sound. The change happens because the larynx, or voice box, is lengthening, and the vocal cords are becoming longer. Every once in a while, voice change can be really obvious. Suddenly, while speaking normally, your voice might "crack" or squeak. The squeak can be embarrassing. While there is little you can do to stop this from happening, the squeaking will eventually end. It just takes time.

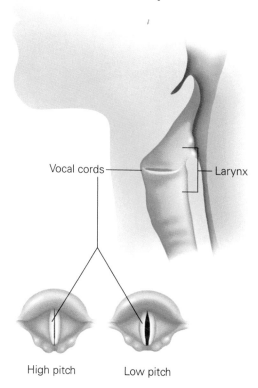

The Larynx

Vocal cords — Larynx

High pitch   Low pitch

The vocal cords are an important part of the larynx. When the cords are open and relaxed, the voice is deeper (low pitch). When the cords are closed and tighter, the voice is higher (high pitch).

Growth Spurts

Growth spurts are periods of sudden and rapid body growth. Growth spurts can seem to happen overnight. They don't really happen that fast, but they are speedy. During a growth spurt, your body grows quickly for a short period of time and then slows down. It is possible to shoot up several centimetres in a short time.

Growth spurts are not just about getting taller. Your body also gains weight and fills out as muscles and bones grow and get stronger.

During growth spurts, you might feel or even act clumsy. That's because your body parts need to catch up to one another, and that takes time. If you are tripping over bigger feet, you are coping until the rest of your body has caught up. Over time, you will feel and be less awkward.

growth spurt: a period of sudden and rapid growth

Keep It Clean

When it comes to puberty, the phrase "keep it clean" refers to more than your language. It refers to a basic fact of life. If a body can sweat, it can smell.

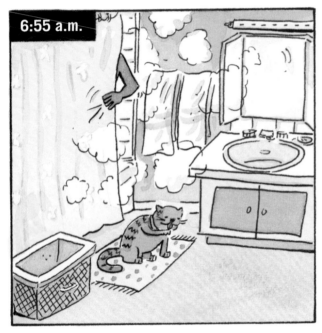

Shower or bathe daily to remove perspiration, bacteria, and dirt. This is a basic step for keeping healthy.

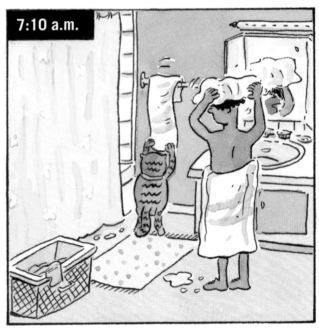

Wash your hair more frequently if it is becoming oily. Conditioner can tame fly-away hair, but overuse can make it seem oily.

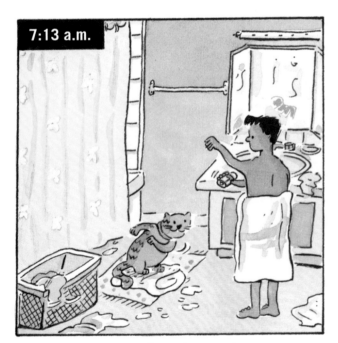

Use a deodorant or antiperspirant under your arms to reduce odour.

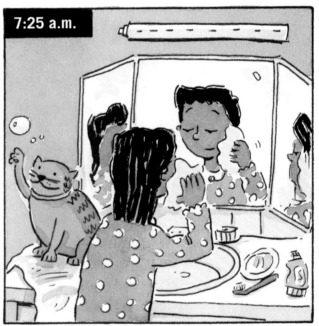

Wash your face gently with soap and water twice daily to take care of oiliness. Don't scrub; this will just irritate your skin and won't make it any cleaner.

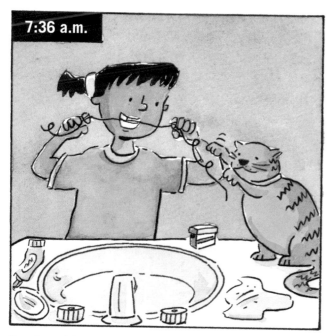

Brush and floss your teeth twice a day, just like always. To help reduce mouth odour and keep your breath fresh, brush your tongue well when you are brushing your teeth—it makes a big difference.

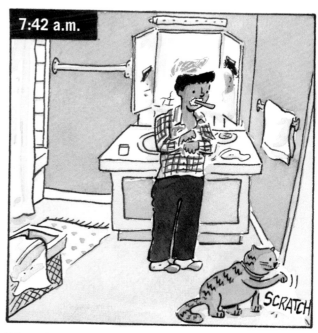

Wear clean clothes, including clean underwear and socks, every day. Why? Because clean clothes do not have old sweat in them. Therefore, they don't smell.

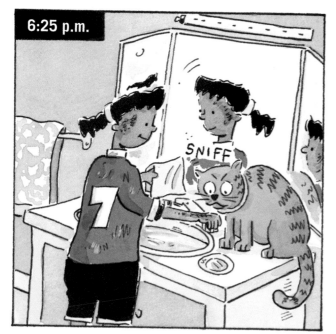

After sports or Phys. Ed. class, wash yourself down. Be sure to wash your face, underarms, feet, and any other areas that perspire. Then dry off and reapply deodorant.

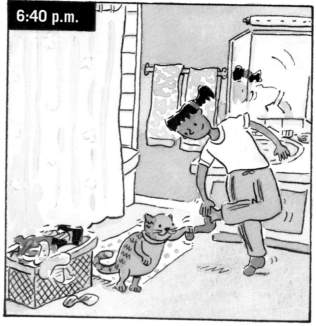

Feet perspire, so remember to wash them well and dry them thoroughly. Put on clean, dry socks after exercise or sports. If your shoes smell, try changing the insole (the inner lining) of each shoe, if it is removable.

Puberty on Your Mind

During puberty, your mind is changing as much as your body is. Your emotions are becoming more complicated and could even be confusing. For example:

- If you felt angry about something before, chances are you are feeling **ANGRY** now.

- If you had hurt feelings before, chances are you are feeling HURT now.

You get the idea—your emotions are heightened. It's almost like your feelings become more "colourful." You are also developing new interests and ideas. You are thinking in new ways and getting better at making choices and solving problems in your life.

Here's a Hint

Questions about puberty are not jokes, and you don't have to feel silly for asking them. If you feel embarrassed or are made to feel silly for asking the questions, find someone else to chat with.

QuickQuiz

Do you ever:

- laugh like crazy about some silly little thing?
- feel like a child sometimes and like an adult at other times?
- get upset easily about little things?
- become furious with someone for no real reason?
- feel confused about how you feel?
- have hurt feelings, more than you used to?
- get embarrassed easily?
- lose your temper?
- worry about how you look?
- feel incredibly happy?

Congratulations! Your emotions are telling you that you are in puberty.

Talking It Over

You may have questions about puberty now, and in the future. Talking with friends can help because they may be experiencing many of the same changes you are. But sometimes friends are not the best source for correct information. Sometimes their information is based on what they think, and not on fact.

Having the wrong information from friends can end up confusing you, or worse, it can lead you to making the wrong choices. And you may end up giving other people that wrong information.

If you have questions about puberty, there are adults who can help you. Choose quiet times to talk about the changes you are going through. You can ask questions or just talk about how things are going and how you are feeling. Parents can be good people to talk to. You may also know other adults, perhaps relatives or friends, who make you feel comfortable and are willing to talk with you.

There are other ways to get information and answers to your questions. You can talk with your Health teacher or any other teacher who makes you feel at ease. Just ask if you could talk for a few minutes in private. Some schools have a counsellor or community health nurse who will be willing to talk with you. You can also talk to your family doctor. Don't forget to use resources such as libraries for books about puberty and adolescence.

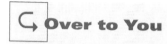

Over to You

Just for You: Sometimes it's hard to start a conversation with an adult when you want to talk seriously. Write the first two sentences you could use to start a serious conversation.

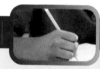

Ask Sam

Dear Sam,

Everybody else is having all these puberty things happening. But me—nothing. When's it going to be? What if it never happens?

Tired of Waiting

Dear Tired of Waiting,

Remind yourself that puberty begins with changes you cannot see, such as the production of hormones.

Puberty can be a frustrating time because you have no control over when things happen. If you can handle the answer: "wait, be patient," that's great, because puberty will happen. But if you are really worried about puberty, it's time to talk with a parent or your family doctor.

Sam

Personal Reflection

When you walk past a mirror, you get a glimpse of yourself. If you stop and look closely for a moment, you get a much better look at your reflection. The same thing happens when you take time to think about yourself. If you take a few quiet minutes to think and reflect, you can get a good idea about who you are and what you are about.

Reflecting about something simply means thinking carefully about it. **Personal reflection** is thinking about yourself and your life— past, present, and future.

Reflecting requires some time alone. You can reflect during any part of your day. A few minutes in the morning or just before going to sleep may be good times. A quiet time is important so remove any distractions, such as TV. Concentrate on you, not on anything else.

Reflection is more than daydreaming. It is active thinking. You may think about something that has just happened and what you can learn from it. You may make plans or imagine yourself in the future.

This is the time to concentrate on yourself in a positive way. This is not a time for fault-finding, blaming, or criticizing yourself. You may think of things that have happened, but remind yourself that this is the time to move forward. Smart people know that having a few minutes to themselves just to think will help them to focus on their goals, gather their strength, and move forward.

personal reflection: serious thoughts you have about yourself and your life

Here's a Hint

Personal reflection can help you gain confidence and prepare you to take on the world. It can be a calming, peaceful moment in a busy day, or it can be an exciting time when you make a plan and know that it is possible. However you use it, when you take time for positive personal reflection, you are doing a healthy thing.

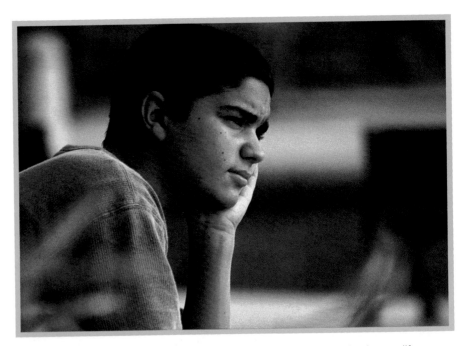

Personal reflection is time you spend thinking about what is happening in your life.

Teen **Consumers**

A **consumer** is someone who buys or uses products. Consumers make decisions each time they spend money. Teens are an important group of consumers, especially of body-care products. Body-care products are all those items we use to clean and enhance our bodies. They include products for skin, teeth, hair, body odour, mouth odour—you get the idea.

Many companies see teens as a **target group,** an important group of consumers that gets special attention because it has money to spend. Companies spend millions of dollars creating advertisements designed especially to appeal to teens.

consumer: someone who buys or uses products

target group: a group of consumers that gets special attention because it has money to spend

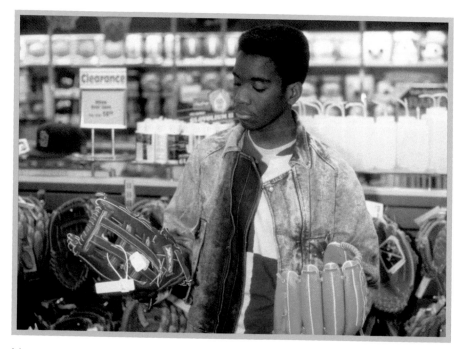

Many advertisements appeal specifically to teens because companies see teens as an important group of consumers.

↳ **Over to You**

Think about advertisements you see on TV, the Internet, or in magazines. Do any of these advertisements use teen models? Do you pay more attention to advertisements that use teens to sell a product? Explain your answer.

The Impact of Advertising

Advertising has a powerful influence on what you choose to buy. The goal of advertising is to short-circuit your thinking so that you don't make a wise choice. Advertisers want you to forget about making a good decision.

Companies use numerous techniques, or methods, in their advertisements so that you will buy their products. The products might be food, clothing, music CDs, body products—anything! These are some of the techniques they use:

- **Music:** The use of familiar music by a popular band or singer.

- **Rewards:** You could get an extra soft drink or a free T-shirt if you buy a certain product.

- **The promise of more personal appeal:** Some advertisements are designed to make you believe that if you buy a particular product, you will be more attractive.

- **Humour:** Sometimes the advertisement uses animals or small children that are cute and funny, or appeals to your sense of humour in other ways.

- **Celebrity endorsements:** Famous people tell you how much they like the product, how it makes them feel and look better.

- **Appeal to emotions:** The advertisement links a story about love, happiness, or friendship to the use of a certain product.

Once you understand the influence of advertising, you can be a smart consumer. Before making your decision ask yourself, "Do I need this item, or is the advertising for it so appealing that it makes me want to buy it now?"

What You Buy

Before you make a decision about what products to buy, you should know how much the product costs. It also helps to ask yourself if you really need the product. Is it essential or is it a luxury? This is a question that sometimes only you can answer.

Here's a Hint

The most important question you can ask yourself before you buy a product is whether you need it, or you just want it. This is a question that sometimes only you can answer.

⟲ Over to You

Create a cartoon or story for a shampoo ad that you think would appeal to students your age. Think about the message you want to send to teens. What technique will you use for your ad?

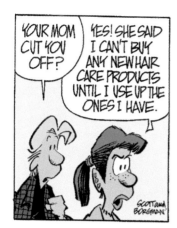
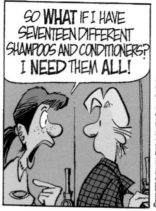
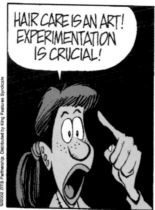
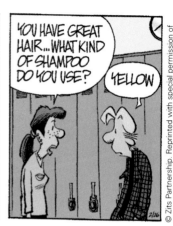

How do you think advertisements have influenced these teens?

Having reliable information about the products you buy is also helpful. Sources of reliable information are around you if you are open to using them. Friends who have tried other body-care products can tell you about them. Informed adults, including your parents and teachers, can also be a good source of information. Sometimes your decision is swayed by the price. If you know that two different brands of the same product do about the same job, you can choose to buy the less expensive one and save money.

Advertising is not a reliable source of information. Some information in the advertisement might be true. For example, shampoo can smell like flowers, antiperspirant can be invisible when you wear it, and gel can set your hair. But shampoo cannot change your personality, antiperspirant does not make you a sports hero, and gel cannot create friends.

⤷ Over to You

1. Make a list of three body-care products that you use. Did advertising influence your decision to use these particular products? Are these products necessities?

2. Find two advertisements you like. Would you buy the products? Do you need the products? Explain.

Making **CHOICES**

Using a PMI Chart

Making a choice can be easy: you can always flip a coin. Making a *wise* choice involves some thought on your part. A choice is usually between two or more possibilities. Before you make a choice about something, you need to have information about each possibility.

Writing down what you know about each possibility is helpful. It allows you to think about all the information you have. You can then compare one possible choice with another.

When you are making consumer choices, it helps to use a PMI chart like the one below.

- The **Plus** column is for all the information you gather that supports making this choice.

- The **Minus** column is for all the information you can think of that is against making this choice.

- The **Interesting Information** column is for information that is neither plus nor minus. It is for any information that is interesting about the choice.

Once you have gathered all this information and thought about it, you can make your choice.

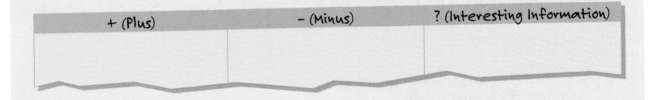

+ (Plus)	– (Minus)	? (Interesting Information)

Fast Fact

To find out the cost per unit, divide the price of the product by the number of units of the product (e.g., milligrams [mg], millilitres [mL], etc.) that the package contains. For example, for a $1.50 tube of toothpaste that contains 130 mL, divide $1.50 by 130.

⤵ Over to You

1. Choose a body-care product that you use. Make a PMI chart for this product. Include information such as the brand, price, availability, how well it works, and other information you would find useful. Figure out how much the product costs per unit.

2. In a store, find two other brands of this product you might want to try. For example, if you use a popular dandruff shampoo, find another two brands of dandruff shampoo. Note the name of each product, the price, and the number of units. It is not necessary to buy the product.

3. Make a PMI chart for these products. Based on the information you have gathered, which brand would you choose? Explain your choice.

Media Influences

Media is a broad term that describes different kinds of communication. Advertising is one kind of media that influences how we think and feel about ourselves. Other media messages come from song lyrics, music videos, TV, movies, magazines, books, Web sites, Internet message boards, and even computer games.

These messages can influence the way we think about ourselves because we tend to compare our appearance and actions with the images we see. The images in the media, however, are usually unrealistic.

Think about the models or stars you see in advertisements or music videos. These people are usually glamorous. They wear beautiful clothes. Their skin is perfect. They seldom wear glasses or have braces or freckles or pimples. Most models are much thinner or more muscular than the average person. They pose or move in suggestive and unnatural ways. In short, these images don't reflect the way real people look and act.

When we compare ourselves to these images, there's a good chance that we feel our bodies don't match the images we see on TV or in advertisements. We can begin to think that we don't look or act the way we should. Our thoughts then influence our feelings—and we may end up feeling negative and unsure about ourselves.

media: different kinds of communication, usually to a large number of people

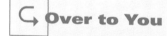

VIP! VERY IMPORTANT POINT

People are unique in the way they look. They come in different sizes and shapes. Most videos and advertisements fail to show just how many different kinds of people there are.

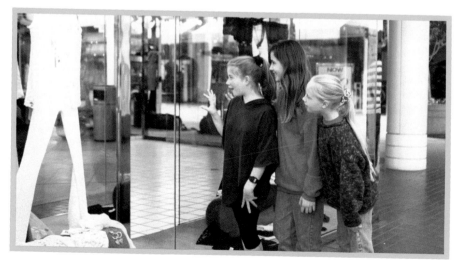

Advertising often uses models who are much thinner and taller than the average person. Most advertisements don't reflect how people really look.

⤷ Over to You

As a class, make a list of three popular TV ads or music videos. Discuss how teens are portrayed in these media. Make a list of what you like and don't like about what these media are saying about teens.

Understanding Body Image

body image: the collection of pictures and thoughts we have in our minds about how our bodies look

Negative thinking about ourselves affects our body image. Our **body image** is the collection of pictures and thoughts we have in our minds about our physical appearance. These personal thoughts can be so hidden that they are often difficult to explain to others. However, this internal image has a big impact on how we feel about ourselves.

A negative body image can leave you feeling less valuable, unimportant, not worthwhile. It can work like a brick wall, stopping you from trying new things and enjoying life. A negative body image can stop you from liking yourself. A positive body image can move you forward. You feel confident and willing to try new things. You enjoy who you are.

A Healthy Body Image

healthy body image: liking who you are

A **healthy body image** is accepting and liking the way you are, "feeling good inside your skin." That means having a positive attitude about your body, your talents, and your personal beliefs. A healthy body helps create a healthy body image.

A healthy body is not necessarily the kind of body we see in the media. A healthy body is one that reflects a balance of healthy eating and physical activity. If you think you have an imbalance, take action. Change one side of the balance. You can create a healthy body image by finding this balance and keeping it. Remember: A healthy body is one that is right for *you*. It does not need to match media images.

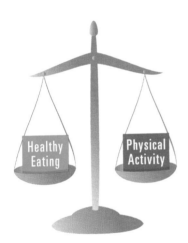

You can create a healthy body image by finding a balance of healthy eating and physical activity—and keeping it.

↳ Over to You

1. a) An advertisement can be so memorable that parts of it stick in your mind. As a class, make a list of as many jingles, tunes, songs, and slogans from advertising that you can recall. Add the name of the product being advertised (if you can remember it).

b) Discuss why you think people remember these jingles, tunes, songs, or slogans. Are there any jingles or slogans you remember, even though you don't remember the actual product being advertised? Do you think advertisers would be pleased to hear this? Why or why not?

c) In Chapter 3, you saw how different factors influence food choices. Discuss at least three ways the media might influence your food choices.

◀◀ Now You Know

→ Puberty is the stage in life when you go from being a child to being an adult. Changes in puberty can occur over several years.

→ Taking some time for personal reflection helps you to better understand how you feel and what you think about yourself.

→ Advertisers target teens because they are an important group of consumers.

→ A smart teen consumer can decide whether an item is needed or just desired.

→ A healthy body image includes a positive attitude about your body, your talents, and your personal beliefs.

↻ Over to You

1. Collect several examples of advertising directed toward teens from a magazine or other print source. Use these examples to create a collage of messages being sent to teens. For example, how they should look, what they should wear, what they like to do. Working in small groups, discuss whether you agree or disagree with the messages. Make a list of messages about teens that you think should be included in advertising. Read your list to the class.

2. Imagine that you and your friends have grown up and live on an island with absolutely no access to advertising or media (that's right, no TV, movies, magazines, or Internet). Describe what you think you and your friends would be like. What do you think you would do for enjoyment? How would you decide what to wear or what to buy? What would you think was important in life?

3. Working in small groups, create a new "teen product." For example, your product could be a face cleanser or a pair of jeans. Write a TV or radio advertisement for this product. Show how you would like to see teens portrayed in your advertisement. Act out the advertisement with a partner or partners.

Key terms

personal values, alternative, consequence, peers, peer pressure, coercion, intimidate, assertive, abuse

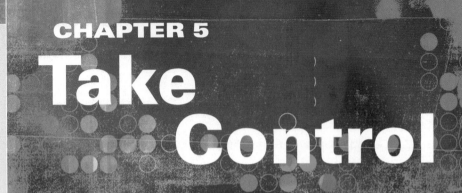

CHAPTER 5
Take Control

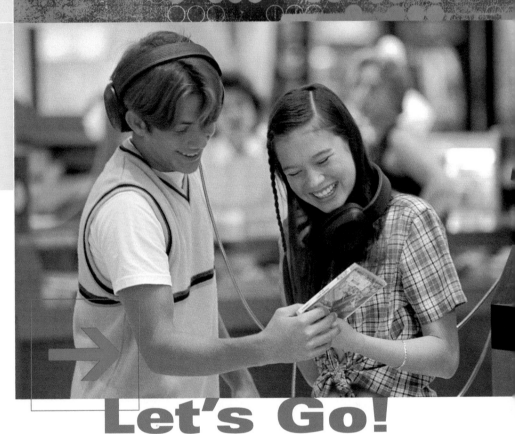

Let's Go!

→ When was the last time you did something simply because your friends were doing it?

→ Have you ever done something you didn't want to do because you were afraid to say "no"?

→ When was the last time a friend said "no" to a suggestion you made?

You make many decisions in your life. Some of these decisions are small and don't take much thought. Others require a lot more attention. There are times when you might decide to do something in order to please someone or to fit in with your group of friends. In certain situations, you might do something because you don't know how to refuse. Sometimes you might be confused about what to say or do.

In this chapter, you will see how different pressures can influence your decisions. You will also see how there are ways of saying "no" to something that you don't want to do.

What Should I Do?

Every day you make many decisions. Some decisions don't have a clear right or wrong answer. For example, should you try out for the soccer or basketball team? The answer would be neither right nor wrong.

Other decisions do have a right and wrong answer. These kinds of decisions test your **personal values,** how you judge what is right and wrong. Whether to cheat on a test, skip school, or smoke a cigarette on a dare are examples of decisions that involve a right and wrong choice.

When you make a decision, you think about the different options, or **alternatives,** available. You also think about the **consequences** of your decision—what will happen when you act on your decision. Then you select the choice that is best for you.

personal values: beliefs that are important to you

alternative: a possibility or option

consequence: the result of an action

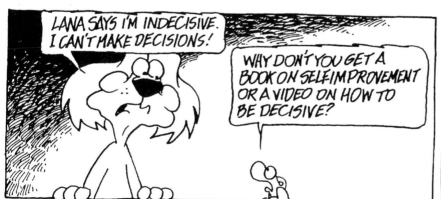

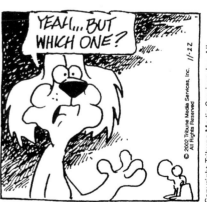

Influences

Many people can influence your decisions. Parents and family are a major influence in your life. Your parents are naturally concerned about your well-being and safety. They know your strengths and weaknesses, and there will be situations where their advice or opinions will help you decide what to do.

Another major influence in your life is your peers. Your **peers** are people who are equal or similar to you in some way. They may be other students in your class. They could be members of your judo class, teammates in sports activities, or members of your music group.

Peers influence you because they do things that appeal to you. Chances are, you want to do these things too. Your peers are important because they help you to discover who you are. When you are with your peers, you can share ideas, activities, and opinions. When you are accepted by your peers, you feel comfortable. You have a sense of belonging and you feel more confident.

⤷ Over to You

1. What are three situations in which you would find your family's advice helpful?

2. Make a web diagram with you in the centre. Show the different groups of people you feel are your peers. Below the diagram, give examples of how these people are like you. What interests do they share with you?

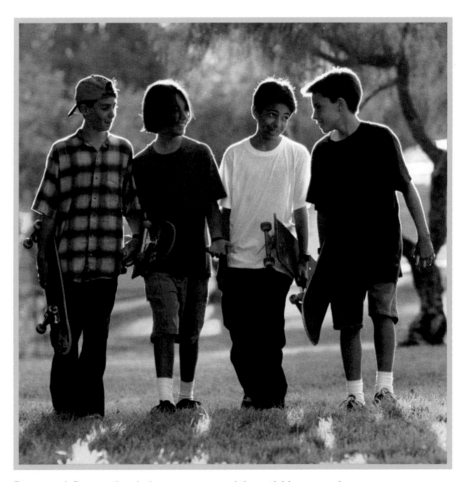

Peers can influence the clothes you wear and the activities you enjoy.

Peer Pressure

Your peers can do more than just influence your decisions. They can pressure you to act a certain way or to become like them. **Peer pressure** is a good thing when it encourages you to participate in healthy behaviour. You might try certain sports or become a member of a club because of the pressure from peers. You also learn important social skills from peers. For example, you have probably learned that bragging turns people off; sharing makes you likeable; and lying to friends is unpopular.

Peers can also pressure you to make unhealthy decisions. They can influence you to do things that you would not usually do on your own. Your peers can make some activities sound attractive, even if they are not safe or legal. Unhealthy decisions make you feel uncomfortable because they go against your personal values.

You Can Pressure Peers Too

Just as peers can pressure you to make certain decisions, the reverse is also true—you can influence the decisions your peers make. You can encourage your peers to try new things and make wise decisions. You can also pressure people to make decisions that are not so wise.

peer pressure: the strong influence to behave in a manner that is acceptable to others

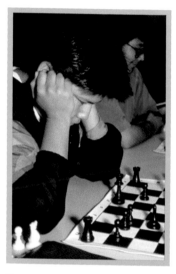

You can encourage your peers to try new activities.

↳ Over to You

1. On your own, list five decisions you have made in the past week. These could be decisions about food, school activities you participated in, movies you saw, or other decisions. What were some alternatives to the choices you made?

2. Discuss your list of decisions and the alternatives with a partner. Which decisions did not have a clear right or wrong answer? Did any decisions involve using your personal values? If so, which ones?

3. **Just for You:** Some friends suggest watching a horror movie that one person doesn't want to see. When this person objects, the others laugh and make fun of this person. The person finally gives in and watches the movie. Have you ever pressured someone to do something he or she did not want to do? Did you tease this person? What was the result?

4. List five ways peers can be a positive influence. Now list five ways peers can be a negative influence.

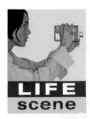

LIFE scene

Pressure

Imagine that you are part of the following scenes. What are you being pressured or encouraged to do in each scene? How would you respond in each situation?

Seb is a really popular guy in your group. He likes to make people laugh. Every time this one student says something in class, Seb raises his eyebrows in disgust. Then he makes a face and looks at you. He expects you to laugh. You don't like what Seb is doing, but you know he'll start making fun of you if you don't go along with him and laugh at the student too.

Claire has been grounded, but she plans to meet her friend at the mall on Saturday afternoon. She has told her mom that she'll be studying at your place that day. Claire asks you to go along with the story if anybody asks you where she is.

Glen has some cigarettes. He offers you one. Two voices start talking in your head. One says, "If I say no, Glen will make fun of me." The other voice says, "I hate the smell of smoke. I really don't want to do this."

You want to start earning money by babysitting, but you don't want to take a babysitting course on your own. Reena calls you to tell you that she and her brother are taking the babysitting course. She wants to know if you want to take the course with them.

Your Math class is writing a unit test. You're halfway through the test when Ben taps you on the shoulder and indicates that he wants you to show him your answers.

Six Steps to Making a Decision

When you make a decision, you usually decide so quickly that you often don't think about what you are doing. Slowing down the process and taking the following six steps can help you make a more informed decision.

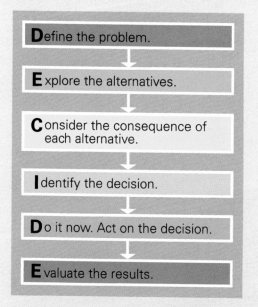

Define the problem.

Explore the alternatives.

Consider the consequence of each alternative.

Identify the decision.

Do it now. Act on the decision.

Evaluate the results.

Let's see how these steps might help you when you are in a difficult situation.

1. **The problem:** Some friends have dared you to send a threatening note to a student in your class. You want to be accepted by this group, but you don't agree with what they want you to do. What should you do?

2. **You have three alternatives:** You could ignore them and hope that they stop pestering you. You could say "no," or you could send the note.

3. **You consider the consequence of each alternative:** If you ignore the group, they could pester you even more. If you say "no," they might stop pressuring you, or they might snub you. If you send the note, you could get caught. You might also feel uncomfortable because you know that it is not the right thing to do.

4. **You identify the decision:** You decide not to send the note.

5. **You act on your decision:** You tell your friends you are not going to send the note.

6. **You evaluate the results:** Your friends call you a "chicken," but you feel you did the right thing. You can put up with the name-calling because you feel good about yourself. You are proud of your decision.

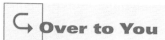

Over to You

With a partner, work through the Six Steps to Making a Decision for the following situation:

You have made a commitment to babysit for your neighbours on Saturday afternoon. It is now Friday. Your friend has an extra ticket to a concert for that afternoon and is inviting you to go. What would you do?

Choice and Coercion

Your friend Nick has asked you four times this week to join the swim team. Your friend Jen keeps asking you to sign up for the 6-km walkathon. You're not sure you want to participate in these activities. In each of these cases, you feel pressure to do something, but what you finally decide to do will be *your choice.* You will have control of the decision.

In some situations, it seems that there is less choice. People can be more forceful in getting you to do something. You feel that you have to do what these people say because you are afraid of what they will do or say if you answer "no." These people are using **coercion** to get you to do something. Coercion is much stronger than peer pressure. You are being coerced if you feel that you can't say "no" because you will be embarrassed, **intimidated,** isolated, or made to feel very uncomfortable in some other way.

coercion: the act of forcing someone to do something that he or she doesn't want to do

intimidate: to frighten someone in order to force that person to do something

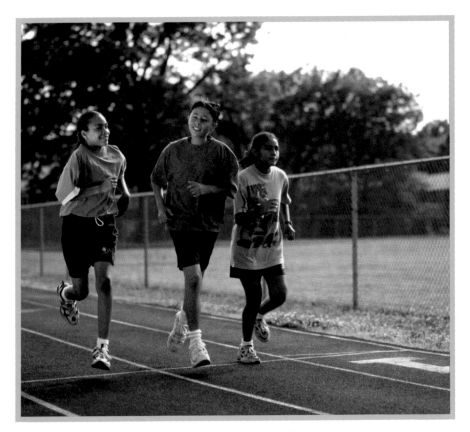

You can make your own choices. You can choose the activities that you want to participate in.

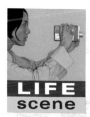

Choice or Coercion: How Does It Feel?

Imagine yourself in each situation described below. How would you feel?

Situation 1

You are standing in the cafeteria line at school during lunch hour. Jamie, a popular student from class, asks you for some money so she can buy a soft drink. You say you don't have any spare change. Jamie insists that you hand over some cash or else she'll make sure everyone knows how "cheap" you are. She tells you she'll yell it out right now in front of everyone. You decide to give Jamie the little money you have so that she doesn't make fun of you in front of the entire cafeteria crowd.

Situation 2

You are standing in the cafeteria line at school during lunch hour. Jamie, a popular student from class, asks you for some money so she can buy a soft drink. You say you don't have any spare change. Jamie moves on to ask the next person in line. You decide that you could probably contribute to Jamie's collection. You call Jamie back to offer her some money.

When you are making a choice, you feel:

- **right about that choice**
- **free to make that choice**
- **in charge of your actions**

When you are being coerced, you do not have these feelings.

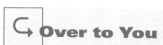

Over to You

Your friend dares you to steal a CD from a music store. Your friend threatens to stop speaking to you if you don't steal the CD. Do you think this is peer pressure or coercion? Explain your answer.

Learning to Say "No"

Saying "no" to someone who is pressuring or coercing you to do something can be difficult. You might need to practise saying "no" on your own a few times. Not every situation will be the same, so having a "tool box" of refusal skills can be helpful. Here are a few tips on how to say "no."

- Walk away. Say nothing, just leave.

- Say "no" or "no, thank you." You don't have to give a reason.

- Suggest doing something else or distract your friends by changing the subject.

- Make an excuse to leave, and walk away.

- Delay. Tell your friends that you might join them later.

- Try being funny. Humour can help relieve tension.

- Find someone in the group who agrees with you. This can give you the strength you need to resist peer pressure.

When you say "no" to someone, be **assertive.** State your position in a clear, confident, and honest way. "I decided not to do that" and "I am going to do this instead" are examples of being assertive. Once you've made your choice, be confident and stick with it. If your friends don't take you seriously, tell them again. Let them know you've made a decision that is *best for you.*

Saying "No" to an Adult

It's hard to say "no" to a peer, but it can be even harder to say "no" to an adult. It is OK to say "no" to an adult if that person is doing something or asks you to do something that makes you feel uncomfortable. For example, if you are concerned about accepting a ride from someone who has been drinking alcohol, tell that person you don't feel comfortable getting into the car. If you have access to a phone, call a parent or someone you trust and arrange for another ride.

Here's a Hint

Saying "no" to someone who is pressuring you to do something is a way of being in control of your actions. Once you say "no," you may also find that others will respect you for your decision.

---

assertive: expressing oneself in a clear, positive, and firm way, without being rude

---

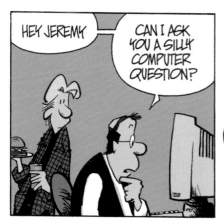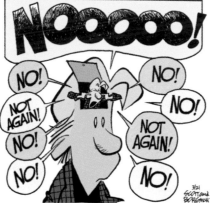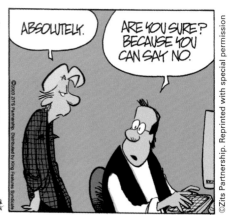

Why does Jeremy say "no" in his head but "absolutely" out loud?

Accepting "No" as an Answer

Just as you might say "no" to some choices that you are offered, your friends might say "no" to some of your suggestions. When someone says "no" to your suggestion, that person is making a personal choice. If people say "no" to you, it does not mean that they don't like you, or that they don't want to be your friend. They just don't want to do what you are doing. Remember: It's OK to be refused.

↳ Over to You

1. Write two words that you think describe someone who uses coercion to get people to do something. Create a cartoon or drawing that illustrates these words.

2. In a small group, create three scenes where someone is being pressured to do something that he or she doesn't want to do. Using the tips on page 66, explain how the person could say "no" in each situation.

3. **Just for You:** Think about a situation where you know you should have refused to do something, but you didn't know how to say "no." What would you do in the same situation now?

Teen Issues: Using Substances

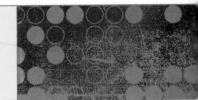

Teens face issues about using cigarettes, alcohol, prescription drugs, legal drugs, illegal drugs, and other substances. How you handle these issues will say a great deal about you. If you are willing to take control of your life and your own actions, then you will be able to make wise decisions about substance use.

Substance Use and Abuse

There are many substances that can be used, and the list is always growing. That's why for now, we are calling everything a "substance." Any time you read the word "substance," you can replace the word with the name of the actual substance you are thinking about. For example, if you are thinking about drinking beer, then use the word "beer" each time you read the word "substance" here. The next time you are thinking about a different substance, use its name instead.

Any substance that can be used can also be **abused.** If a substance is used for the wrong reason, if the wrong amount is taken, or if it is used in the wrong way, the substance is being abused. The user is making an unhealthy decision. Some substances are illegal for everyone; others are illegal only for certain groups.

abuse: to use improperly

Prescription Medicine

Prescription medicine is medication that can be obtained only with a doctor's permission. Antibiotics, insulin, and strong painkillers are examples of prescription drugs.

Prescription medicine is safe only for the person who gets the prescription from the doctor. It is dangerous to use another person's medicine. It is also dangerous to use your own medicine in ways not prescribed by a doctor.

Fast Fact

Young athletes may get offered substances that increase strength artificially. Many of these substances are illegal. Using some of these substances is considered cheating. All these substances are dangerous to your health.

Why Some Teens Use or Abuse Substances

It has been said that there are as many reasons for using substances as there are people. It is true that each person has his or her own reasons for using any substance. A person might give some of these reasons:

- I want to be liked.

- I want to fit in.

- Other people might make fun of me—or worse—if I don't go along with the group.

- I'm curious. I want to try it because I have seen other people doing it.

- Everyone's doing it.

- It looks "cool."

- It makes me happy.

- It takes my mind off other things, off everything.

- It is a great escape.

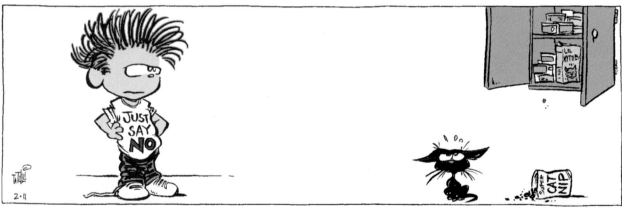

Drugs have consequences. If you have questions, talk to someone who can help, such as a parent, teacher, or guidance counsellor.

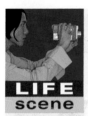

LIFE scene

It's All Substance Abuse

In the following scenes, teens have chosen to abuse substances.

A 13-year-old boy takes beers from the fridge in his parents' home. He drinks them alone in his room and then hides the empty bottles until he can sneak them into the garage. His dad wonders why his beer supply is decreasing so fast these days.

A mother comes home to her daughter and her daughter's girl-friend. The two girls are giggly and they have red, irritated eyes. They say their eyes are red because they've been chopping onions for supper. When the mother walks past her daughter's bedroom, she gets a whiff of an odd smell.

A 14-year-old boy picks up his friend at his home on the way to school. The friend hands over two pills. The pills are the friend's prescription drugs. The boy says, "Thanks!" Then he swallows the capsules with a drink from his water bottle.

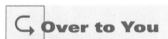

Over to You

From what you have learned, what advice would you offer each teen in the above Life Scene?

Advice and Assistance

If something about your decision is bothering you or you're finding it really difficult to face heavy pressure, then it's time to talk to someone. Talk to a parent, teacher, guidance counsellor, or any other adult you think will listen and help. Talk about how you are feeling. Talk about how you wanted to give in to the pressure and how difficult it was to resist. Or talk about how you did give in but you don't want to make the same decision again. Being in control also means choosing to get advice and assistance when you need it.

Taking Control by Taking Action

If you are willing to take action, you can deal with the pressures to use substances. Any time you find yourself in a situation where you need to make a decision about using a substance, you can be in control by taking these actions:

Stop	You don't have to make a quick decision. If you are being pushed to decide too quickly, then choose "no."
Think	Ask yourself, "Does this feel wrong? Is it illegal? Do I really want to do this? How important is my friends' approval?"
Consider	Imagine the consequences. What will happen if you do this? Consider your reputation. Good or bad, your reputation sticks with you for a long time. What do you want to be known for? What do you want to have other people think about you?
Listen	What is your conscience telling you? If something inside you says "no," if warning bells ring, or if you think you are going to feel bad afterward, don't do it.
Remind Yourself That You Have Choice	Instead of using substances, you can choose to do things that boost you as a person. Substance use does not contribute to who you are or who you want to be.
Decide and Act	Decide what you are going to do and then act on it. Tell people what you have decided. You don't have to explain your reasons. Let people know that you have made a decision that is *best for you*.
Evaluate Your Choice	How do you feel about your decision? Would you make the same choice again?

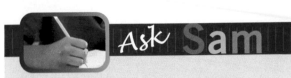

Dear Sam,

I'm in Grade 7, and last Friday night my friend and I went to a dance at the Rec Centre. We were hanging out on the bleachers when some students from Grade 9 came over to talk to us. They said they were going out to smoke some "weed" and asked us to join them. We were flattered that someone in Grade 9 would even talk to us, but we really don't want to do drugs. We didn't know what to do, so we told them we had to go to the bathroom. Now we're feeling kind of foolish. What should we do if this happens again?

Feeling Foolish

Dear Feeling Foolish,

Bravo! You and your friend did the right thing—you walked away from drugs. I can understand how you're feeling now, but how would you feel if you had done something you really didn't want to do? If you rehearse a response now, you will have an easier time saying "no" the next time you are being pressured to do something that makes you feel uncomfortable. To rehearse, do these things:

- Think ahead. Try to predict problems that you might face.

- Decide in advance what you are going to do.

- Think of ways to handle the situation if it happens. And think of some ways to totally avoid the situation.

- Practise with a friend or rehearse by using a mirror. Go over some ways to say "no" in a firm, not hostile, way.

When the time comes, you can respond with words that you've already prepared for such an occasion.

Hope this helps.

Sam

◀◀ Now You Know

→ You make decisions every day. Some decisions involve thinking about your personal values.

→ When you make a decision, you need to think about what will happen when you act on it.

→ Peers are important to your growth and development as an individual. Peers can encourage you to take healthy actions.

→ Peers can pressure you to make unhealthy decisions.

→ You can also pressure your peers to make healthy or unhealthy decisions.

→ You can learn how to say "no." There are different ways of saying "no" to someone who is pressuring you to do something that you don't want to do.

↳ Over to You

1. On your own, think of three situations where you could pressure a friend to do something positive. What would you say to convince your friend to act in each situation? Share this information with a partner.

2. Search magazines to find two or three advertisements for alcohol. Or recall two or three advertisements for alcohol that you have seen on TV or heard on the radio. What message is each advertisement sending about people who drink? What possible consequences of drinking alcohol are not included in the advertisement?

3. With a partner, create a TV or radio advertisement that tells teens how to handle peer pressure or coercion in a positive way. Come up with a slogan that deals with handling pressure from peers. Act out or tape-record your advertisement and present it to the class.

4. Write a poem, song, or rap that describes how to be assertive.

Key terms

physical safety,
precautions, social safety,
emotional safety,
risky behaviour,
personal safety limits,
harassment, bullying,
resilient

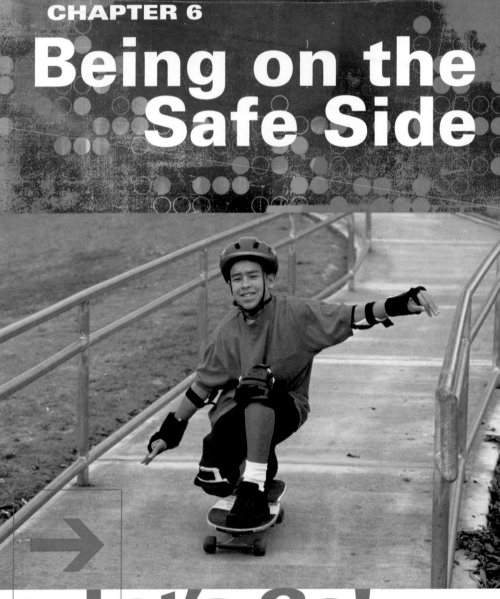

CHAPTER 6
Being on the Safe Side

Let's Go!

→ In your notebook, quickly list 12 safety tips for any areas of your life. Need a hint? Think about being safe at home, at school, in sports, and in other physical activities. Think about times when you are alone and when you are with friends.

→ Compare your list with that of a partner. How do the lists differ? How are they the same? Add any tips from your partner's list that you may not have mentioned.

Being Safe

When you say you are "safe," what comes to mind? Do you mean that you have very few dangers in your surroundings? Do you mean that you are prepared for an emergency? Do you mean that you can handle any person in any situation? In this chapter, you will learn that all of these things are part of being safe.

Personal Safety

Being safe involves many things. It involves being aware of your surroundings. It involves not getting into situations that you think could be dangerous. And it involves knowing at what point you no longer believe you are safe.

There is always something more to learn about your own personal safety. This is good news because the safer you are, the more freedom you have to be the person you choose to be.

Physical Safety

Physical safety means being safe from physical harm. It means protecting your body from hurt or injury. It also means being safe from physical things you can see, such as intersections, the bottom of a cliff, and the bottom of a swimming pool. Physical dangers are the easiest to see, so there are many hints and tips for being physically safe. There are also many **precautions** you can take to be physically safe.

Fast Fact

Some houses in your neighbourhood may have a sign in the window that says **Block Parent.** This sign means that you can go to this house for assistance if you need it. Just explain your situation to the person who lives there and ask for help.

physical safety: protection from danger, physical harm, or injury to the body

precautions: actions a person takes to reduce risk and to be more safe

---

QuickQuiz

What precautions would you take in the following situations?

- A stranger knocks on the door. Your parents aren't home yet.

- You are several blocks from your house, and you think someone is following you.

- You are at your friend's cottage, and she suggests that you both go for a boat ride.

- You and a friend have signed up for racquetball lessons.

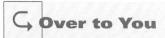

Over to You

Just for You: Make a list of five precautions you take to protect yourself when you play sports or do daily physical activities.

Social Safety

Social safety is the sense of being safe with others. In a socially safe setting, you feel secure, cared for, and trusted. Social safety means you are valued and accepted by your group. You are free to express your ideas, thoughts, and personality, without fear of being laughed at, teased, harassed, or excluded.

Emotional Safety

Emotional safety is when you are aware of your emotions, and you are free to express them in a positive and confident way. If you are emotionally safe, you are not afraid to say "no." You are able to deal with actions and comments that are meant to hurt your feelings. You trust your personal values and beliefs. You are recognized as an individual. And you are proud of who you are.

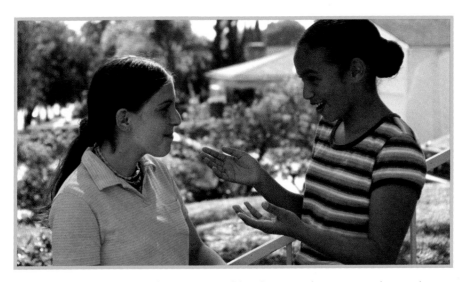

When you are emotionally safe, you are confident in expressing your emotions and thoughts to others.

↳ Over to You

1. Give an example of a time when you were not comfortable sharing your ideas. Why were you uncomfortable? What would you do next time so that you are more comfortable expressing your ideas?

2. What are three things you and your peers can do to improve personal safety in your community and school?

Workplace Safety

Young people can be injured on the job. When you get a part-time job, ask your employer what you should do in case of an emergency and whom you should talk to if you have safety questions. And wear safety equipment, such as the following:

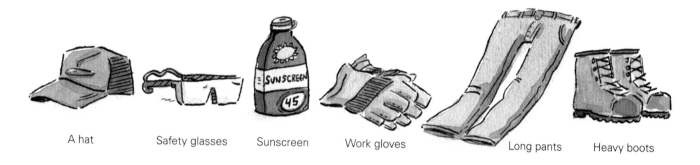

| A hat | Safety glasses | Sunscreen | Work gloves | Long pants | Heavy boots |

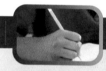

Ask Sam

Dear Sam,

I'm kind of a shy person. I don't feel comfortable talking to people I don't know. It is easier for me to talk with strangers on-line than to talk to people in person. When I'm on-line, I feel at ease asking people for help with my homework and I enjoy just "chatting" with other teenagers. My teacher told me to be careful when I'm on the Internet. She said I need to know how to "surf safely." How can I make sure that I'm safe on the Internet?

Like to Chat

Dear Like to Chat,

You need to take precautions, especially when you are using chat rooms. The most important precaution you can take when you use the Web is to remain anonymous.

Keep all your private information—name, phone number, address, parents' names, passwords, and photos—to yourself. Using a nickname in chat rooms is a good idea. Remember: People can make up anything in a chat room. They might not be telling you the truth about themselves. And don't open files or documents from people you do not know. Just delete these e-mails and tell an adult right away.

Sam

Risky Behaviour

risky behaviour: taking an action when the consequences of the action are not known

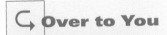

Over to You

With a partner, brainstorm a list of four situations that involve a positive risk. Explain how these risks are positive.

personal safety limits: your line between what you think is safe and what you think is unsafe

How safe you are depends on whether you participate in **risky behaviour.** Each person has his or her own idea of what risky behaviour looks like. What looks or sounds risky to you may not be considered risky by someone else. When you take a risk, you do something without knowing what the consequences of this activity will be.

Some risks are positive because they challenge you to do better and achieve something. Positive risks give you the chance to reach your potential. Other risks are unhealthy, and taking them can be harmful, even dangerous.

When you are deciding whether to take a risk, you need to pay attention to what you think and know and how you feel about the situation. You can control the situation more easily if you establish your own safety limits. Your **personal safety limits** tell you when you are comfortable and when you start to feel nervous, afraid, or uncomfortable.

Everyone has the right to set his or her own safety limits. Learning to tell people about your safety limits is important. It is OK to tell someone that you don't want to do something. You can let people know when you do not feel safe. You can also create safety limits that help to protect you emotionally. For example, you might decide to tell someone that you don't like it when he or she teases you about something.

Some risks are challenges that help you feel better about yourself. If you enter a competition, for example, you might not win, but you will gain confidence from the experience.

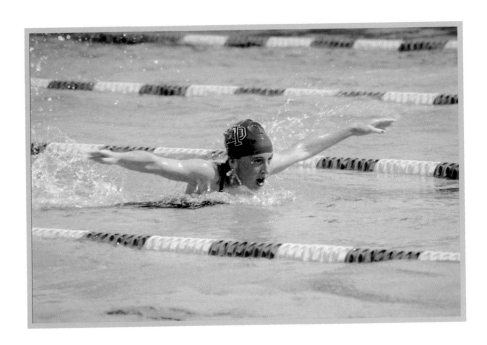

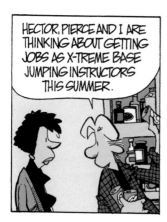
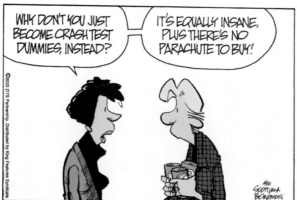
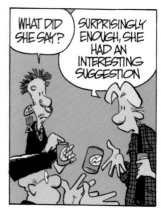

What risks would Jeremy be choosing to take in his summer job?

Measuring Risky Behaviour

A good way to measure a risk is to ask yourself the following questions:

- Why am I taking this risk?

- What will happen if this risk doesn't work out?

- Will I get hurt?

- Will others get hurt?

- What other choices can I make?

⤷ Over to You

1. a) In your notebook, write the risks associated with these activities:

   i) playing volleyball

   ii) smoking cigarettes

   iii) starting a new school

   iv) spreading a rumour

   v) trying some pills that are not yours

   vi) learning to cook

   vii) following fad diets

   viii) applying for a part-time job

b) Compare your answers with those of a partner. Are they the same or different? Explain why.

2. As a class, discuss the kinds of jobs teens can have. Make a list of the possible safety risks in each job.

3. To get information on safety tips for young workers, use a search engine to find the Canadian Centre for Occupational Health and Safety on-line and follow the links.

Harassment

Personal safety limits can help you let other people know what your boundaries are, but sometimes people ignore your limits. They bother you. They say or do things that make you feel angry, embarrassed, or frightened. When people repeatedly act this way toward you, they are harassing you. Even if people tell you that they are "just joking," if what they are doing disturbs you, it is still **harassment.**

The kind of harassment you probably know most about is **bullying.** Harassment, including bullying, is about power. When someone harasses, he or she wants to have power over others in order to make them change their behaviour or feel bad about themselves. People can use many actions to harass others. The table below lists some of these actions.

harassment: the act of tormenting or bothering someone repeatedly

bullying: pressuring people to do something by making them fearful

Harassment	Action
Verbal	• making threats • making rude remarks or telling rude jokes • making comments about a person's religion, clothing, culture, appearance, or gender • spreading rumours about a person • leaving offensive or intimidating phone messages
Physical	• pushing, shoving • blocking a person's way • giving unwanted touching, patting, or pinching • giving any other unwanted physical contact
Visual	• sending someone rude e-mails, photographs, drawings, or cartoons • displaying objects that are offensive
Retaliation	• taking revenge on someone because that person complained about being harassed

Sexual harassment means harassing someone in a sexual way. Sexual harassment can be any of the actions listed above.

Effects of Harassment

If you are being harassed, you can feel helpless. You might think that there is nothing you can do to stop it. You might even blame yourself for what is happening to you. You might also:

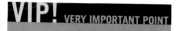

- fear revenge if you take action

- drop activities and avoid going where the harasser might be

- lose your self-confidence

- lose interest in school and activities you enjoy

- develop headaches or feel sick

Because being harassed can really affect your life, you need to take action to end the harassment.

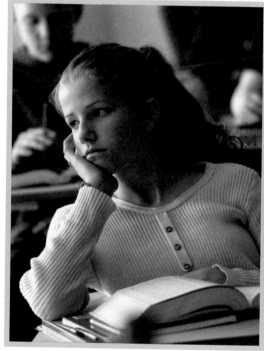

Don't just worry about being harassed. Keeping it a secret will stop you from getting the help you need to end the problem.

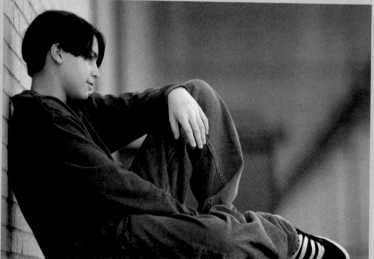

Dealing With Harassment

Ignoring harassment won't always make it go away. If you are disturbed by the cruel way a person is treating you or someone else, you have the right and the responsibility to do something about it.

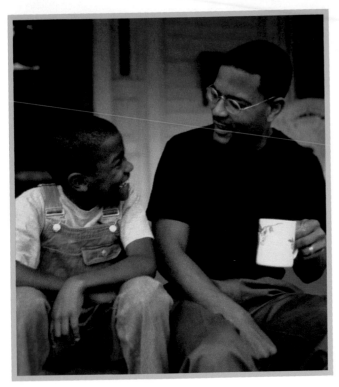

Decide to take action to help yourself. Tell someone who can put an end to the problem.

Here are some actions you could take if you are being harassed or bullied:

- Don't give in to the harasser's demands. Walk away.

- Walk to and from school with a friend or other people.

- Avoid being an easy target—don't go where bullies hang out.

- Keep a record of the incidents (dates, times, places, and witnesses).

- If the harassment continues, find and talk to an adult at school who will help you deal with this problem.

If you have a friend who is being harassed, you can help. You can support your friend by listening and by helping him or her report the incident.

Bullying

❋ Bullies are harassers. They usually pick on others when teachers, parents, or other adults are not around.

❋ People are bullied simply because they are different in some way from the person bullying them.

❋ Bullies seldom work alone. Other students are often aware of the problem. They might encourage the bully to continue. They might simply watch the bully's actions, without doing anything to help the victim. These other people contribute to bullying if they don't do anything to stop it.

❋ It is important to say something and stick up for the person being bullied. This is the only way bullies know they do not have support for what they are doing.

❋ Bullies often get away with their cruel behaviour because people are afraid to tell others what is going on. Sometimes victims fear that the bully might try to "get even." Reporting incidents is not tattling—it's reporting hurtful behaviour.

Solving Problems

When you solve a problem, you try to find a solution that works. Some steps for solving a problem are similar to those for making a decision. When you solve a problem, however, you may have to *create* your own solution. The next time you have a problem, work it through using the following steps.

1. Define the problem.

2. Brainstorm possible solutions. This step requires creative and positive thinking.

3. Consider the consequences of each solution.

4. Choose the solution you think will work best.

5. Do whatever you have to do to make the solution work.

6. Evaluate your solution. Was it the best one? What would you do differently next time?

1. **The problem:** Some girls from your class have been sending you nasty e-mails.

2. **You brainstorm solutions:** You could ignore the e-mails; you could respond to the e-mails and tell the girls to stop harassing you; you could report the incident to your parents.

3. **You consider the consequences:** If you ignore the e-mails, they may or may not stop. If you respond to the e-mails, the girls might stop harassing you, or they might harass you even more. If you tell your parents, the girls could try to get even.

4. **You choose the solution you think will work best:** You decide to respond to the e-mails and deal with the problem.

5. **You do what it takes:** You send an e-mail telling the girls to stop harassing you; you tell your parents what you are doing.

6. **You evaluate your solution:** The e-mails stop. You are happy with your solution.

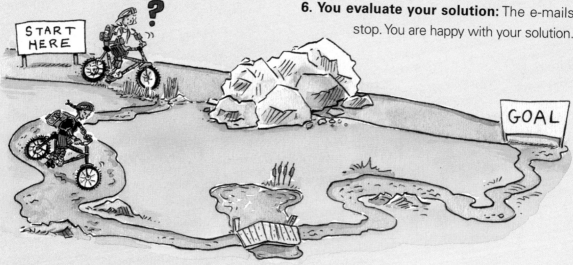

One way to solve a problem is to move around an obstacle that is in your path.

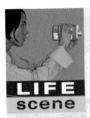

It's All Harassment

Read the following three scenes. Identify what is happening in each scene. What suggestions would you offer to the teens in these situations?

Jun

has just moved to Canada. He doesn't speak much English. A group of boys corner him in the washroom and demand that he hand over his lunch money. They shove him around and tell him he'd better be careful on his way home from school.

Leanne

hangs around with a group of girls who are very popular at school. One night they have a sleepover at her place. One of the girls, Cleo, starts to talk about a new girl in their class. Cleo says she heard that this new girl was expelled from her old school for smoking in the washroom. Leanne knows this rumour is not true.

Terry

is playing baseball. It's his turn at bat. He swings and misses, and eventually strikes out. Terry's team loses the game. That night, Terry receives an e-mail from a teammate telling him that he's not wanted on the team and should "quit or else."

⤷ Over to You

1. **Just for You:** Have you ever seen a bully in action? What did you do? What could you have done? Do you think that doing something would have affected the actions of the bully or the victim? If so, how?

2. With a small group, create a role play showing how the bystander in a bullying situation can become a positive participant by standing up for a peer and stopping the bullying.

3. Each province and territory has laws that protect people from harassment. Find out about the human rights laws where you live. Discuss the findings as a class.

Resiliency

Why is it that some people are able to bounce back from hardships or tragedy more easily than others? They seem to know how to get through almost impossible situations or challenges. People who know how to rise above very difficult situations are **resilient.** They don't give up. They adapt to change. They expect to find a way to have things turn out well. They learn from their mistakes and past experiences.

Being physically and emotionally safe is critical for being resilient. A sense of safety makes you more willing to take risks. When you fail at something or when something tragic happens in your life, taking positive risks is necessary for you to learn and grow. Knowing that you have the support of family, friends, teachers, and other adults gives you the confidence you need to make wise decisions and take positive actions.

resilient: having the personal strength to rise above difficult circumstances and adapt to new situations

People who are resilient are confident in their abilities to overcome obstacles. They think positively.

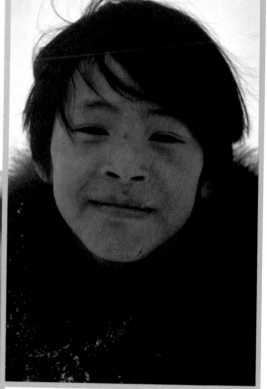

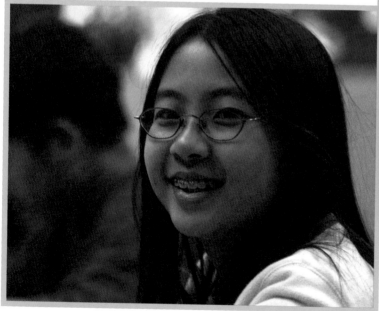

QuickQuiz

How Resilient Am I?

In your notebook, rate yourself from 1 to 5 (1 = Need Work, 5 = Doing Great) on each of the following statements:

1. I have set boundaries for myself so I know when to stop before I do something I don't want to do.
2. I accept responsibility for what I do.
3. Most of the time, I expect things to work out well.
4. I can find someone to help me when I need help.
5. I set goals for myself.
6. I don't get upset when things don't always go my way.
7. I like myself and I am confident in my abilities.
8. When I have a problem, I work to solve it.
9. I don't give up easily.
10. I know that I matter in this world.
11. I know I am not the cause of many problems around me.
12. I have people in my life who love me, no matter what.
13. People generally like me and like to be with me.
14. I am flexible and can handle not knowing how a situation will turn out.
15. I am able to be co-operative and work with others.
16. I can let go of my anger or disappointment and not dwell on it.
17. I like to help others.
18. I learn from my experiences and the experiences of others.
19. I like to laugh and have fun.

Scoring: The higher your overall score, the more resilient you are likely to be. If your score is not that great, don't worry; you can learn to be more resilient.

◀◀ Now You Know

→ Being safe is not just about avoiding physical dangers. You can be safe in physical, social, and emotional ways.

→ You can protect yourself on a job by always wearing the proper protective equipment and learning about the hazards of your job.

→ Whenever you take risks, you learn more about yourself. Risks can be positive, but

you need to set limits to avoid doing something that is unsafe.

→ If you are being harassed or bullied, you must keep telling people what is happening to you until you get help to stop the harassment or bullying. This is not a time to be silent.

→ Resiliency is the personal strength to spring back from difficult experiences and adapt to new situations.

↻ Over to You

1. What is one sport or activity that you like to do? Explain the risks in this sport or activity and how you deal with these risks.

2. Create a poster that shows one characteristic of resiliency.

3. With a partner, research a person who overcame a major problem in his or her life. Make a video or an audio tape in which you and your partner explain who the person is and how he or she overcame the obstacle.

4. Do some research on one of the following programs in your school or community. Develop a short presentation about the

program and its purpose. Present your findings to a group of your peers or a group of younger students in your school.

- Block Parent Program
- peer support groups
- teen self-defence programs
- school patrols
- community police programs
- teen hotlines
- the Alateen program

Key terms

thinking pattern,
confidence, all or nothing,
overgeneralization,
perfectionism,
stress

CHAPTER 7
Feelings

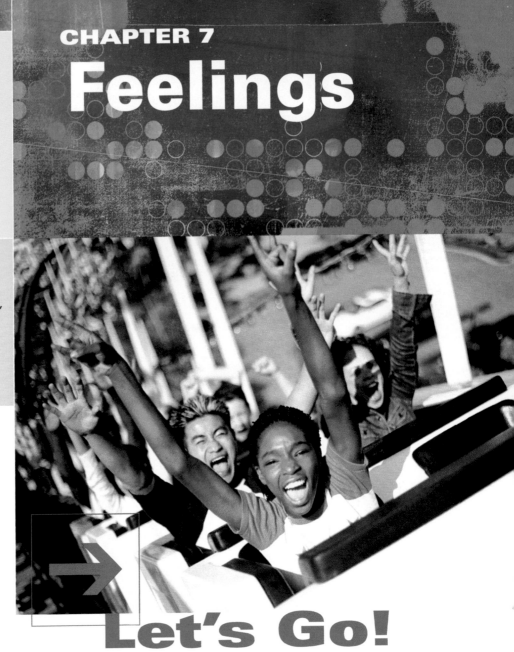

Let's Go!

"Teen emotions are like a roller-coaster ride. It's hard to know what is coming up next."

→ Do you agree with this statement? Why or why not?

→ Do you think your feelings are sometimes like a roller-coaster ride, a speeding race car, or a canoe on calm water? Choose one of these images, or one of your own, to explain your emotions. Give examples from your own experiences to explain your choice.

Thoughts and Emotions

Our thoughts and feelings are closely linked. What we think about a situation can influence how we feel about it.

The relationships you have with other people are also influenced by your thoughts and feelings. Sometimes relationships can make you feel stressed. At these times, you need support and care from others. There will also be times when you can give care and support to someone. In this chapter, you will examine the connection between your thoughts and feelings. You will also explore sources of support that can help you when you need it.

Thinking Patterns

Do you see half a glass of water as "half full" or "half empty"? A person who sees the glass as half full sees something in the glass. For this person, having something in the glass is better than an empty glass. In other words, the situation is positive.

A person who sees the glass as half empty sees something missing from the glass. This person sees something wrong with the situation. This view is a more negative one.

People who see the glass as half full usually have a more positive outlook on life. People who see the glass as half empty usually have a more negative outlook. These outlooks are different thinking patterns. A **thinking pattern** is the way you usually look at a situation and try to understand it.

thinking pattern: the most common way a person thinks about something and explains it

Whenever you face a new situation, your mind jumps into action and starts to explain it to you. Your usual thinking pattern takes over. You can choose whether you have a more positive or more negative thinking pattern.

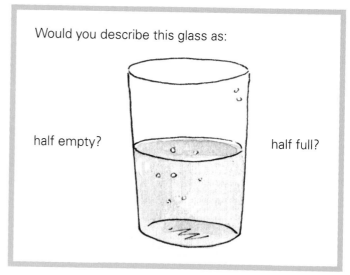

Would you describe this glass as:

half empty?

half full?

Positive Thinking

Because your thoughts and feelings are connected, the way you explain a situation to yourself will influence how you feel about it. If you use a positive thinking pattern, you will feel as if you have a positive attitude. You will then be able to act with a positive attitude, and other people will notice. A positive attitude can give you **confidence** in yourself, in what you think, and in what you do. This belief in yourself, that you are capable and can be trusted, will open doors. You will be able to find new solutions to problems and try new things.

confidence: a belief that you are capable and can be trusted

Here's a Hint

Positive self-talk and visualizations are two important tools for positive thinking. Use them to remind yourself of your talents and what makes you a unique individual.

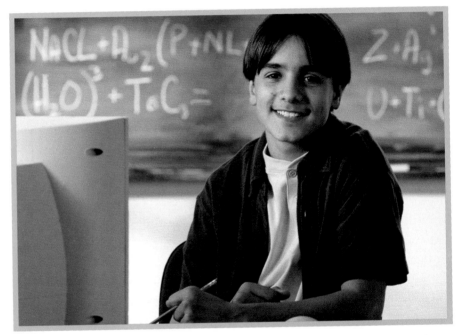

A positive attitude enhances how you view yourself and how you view life in general.

It Is All Connected

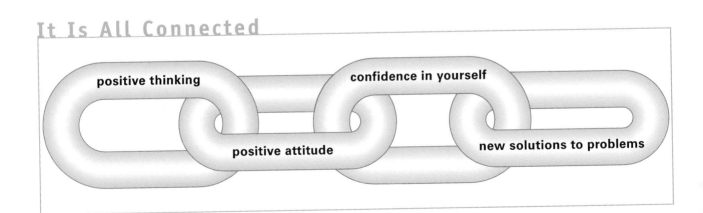

positive thinking — positive attitude — confidence in yourself — new solutions to problems

Not-So-Positive Thinking

Negative thinking and a negative outlook on life can limit who you are. This happens because your negative thoughts do not allow for new ideas and actions. A negative outlook keeps you from having confidence in yourself. Below are some examples of negative thinking patterns.

All or Nothing

When you have an **all or nothing** thinking pattern, you see things as "good" or "bad," "right" or "wrong." There is no in-between. For example, do you ever find yourself thinking, "We play by my rules or else I won't play" or "What I think is right and if you don't agree with me, you're wrong"? This is an all or nothing way of thinking. This thinking pattern keeps you from understanding other people's points of view.

all or nothing: a pattern of thinking where only your own actions or opinions are acceptable to you

Overgeneralizations

Have you ever felt as though *everyone* is picking on you? That *no one* understands you? That you *never* do anything right? When you generalize about situations, you expect the same outcome again and again. When you do this to extremes, you are **overgeneralizing.** You see one problem and think that same problem will always happen. You refuse to think that things could be different. People who generalize use words such as *all the time, everyone, no one, never, every time,* and *always*.

overgeneralization: thinking that is limited by accepting only one possible result, usually a negative one

Perfectionism

Do you believe you must do everything perfectly? Would you say, "If I don't get 100 per cent on this assignment, I'm no good at it"?

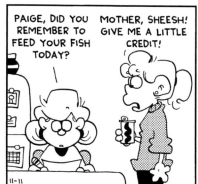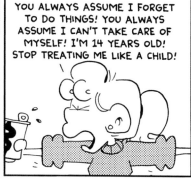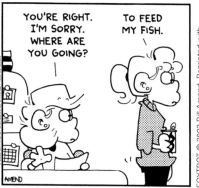

What thinking pattern is Paige using?

perfectionism: a pattern of thinking where a person is not content unless everything is done without any mistakes

Perfectionism is the kind of thinking that makes a person set unreasonable or unrealistic goals. This can lead to great disappointments. If you set your goals so high that you don't turn in assignments because you can't get them "just right," you may be trying to be "too perfect." Do your best and then accept it. Everybody makes mistakes. Mistakes help us to learn other ways of handling a situation.

Luckily, you can decide to change these negative thinking patterns. First, you need to recognize that you are thinking in a negative way. Once you know this, you can break the pattern by substituting positive thoughts for negative ones. This change doesn't happen all at once, but if you remember to use just one or two positive thoughts, you will see a small difference in the way you think. You can then improve your outlook by adding even more positive thoughts when tackling an issue. In time, you will have new ways of looking at many things. Examine the table below and see how thoughts can affect feelings.

Here's a Hint

When you make a mistake or fail at something, ask yourself, "What did I learn from this experience?" Just one answer to this question can make you feel better.

Thoughts and Feelings

	Problem or Situation	Explanation to Self	Feeling
René	• doesn't understand his homework	• "It's the teacher's fault." • "I'm no good in math."	• frustrated • wants to give up
Chris	• does well in music exam	• "I'm a good musician."	• proud, happy
Janie	• scores a goal	• "I played well. Saturday's practice was worth it."	• confident, encouraged

↻ Over to You

1. **Just for You:** Using the table above as a guide, write three examples of problems that you have had or situations that you have been in. How did you explain these to yourself? How did you feel?

2. Explain how thoughts affect feelings.

3. You can choose to have a positive or negative outlook when you think about any situation. Write an example of a positive way to look at the following situations:

   a) You can see your friend only one day this weekend.

   b) You have saved half of the money you need to buy something you really want.

Making CHOICES

Thinking Positively

Negative thought patterns affect your emotions. They also affect your attitude. When you *think* that everyone is picking on you, or that you aren't good enough at something, you start to *feel* negative about yourself. And feeling negative makes you moody. That's when it's time to turn negative thoughts into positive ones.

Use the following steps to help you to turn negative thoughts into positive ones:

1. Identify what is bothering you.

2. Think about what you are telling yourself now. ("I can't do this." "It's my brother's fault." "I give up." "I don't care.")

3. Identify the thought pattern you are using.

4. Figure out how the situation or problem is making you feel. Do you feel angry, lonely, sad, or guilty?

5. Begin to turn negative thinking into positive thinking by making positive statements about how you can deal with the situation.

For example:

"I can't do this."

"I don't care what happens."

"I never do well in ~~track and field~~ art."

↳ Over to You

Apply the steps for positive thinking to the following situations. Write out each step the person can take that will lead to positive thinking.

- Jay is a Grade 7 student who likes drawing and painting. Three weeks ago he entered a school contest. Everyone who entered the contest had to create a poster on safety. Jay felt sure he would win first prize, a CD player. He didn't win. At first he pretended he didn't care, that he thought the contest was "silly." Then he felt angry. Jay didn't hand in any more art assignments. He said he just didn't feel like drawing.

- Anil is playing a quiz game with her family. She usually does very well at the game, but today it seems that every time it is her turn, she doesn't know the answer. She starts to lose the game. She gets angry and leaves the room, telling everyone that she is not playing any more because her questions are harder than everyone else's and it isn't fair.

Stress in Relationships

Because relationships involve at least two people who have their own thoughts and opinions, there are bound to be times of **stress.** Here are some causes of stress in relationships:

- ending a friendship

- dealing with the illness or injury of a family member

- fighting with a friend or someone at school

- arguing with your parents

- having trouble with a sibling

- witnessing arguments between your parents

Over to You

Create a poster or computer screen saver that gives one hint for handling stress in a relationship.

Other changes in a relationship can cause stress. Maybe a close friend starts hanging around with different people because she feels that the two of you don't have much in common any more. Or perhaps your friend doesn't come over to visit as much as he used to because he is spending more time with someone else. In some cases, relationships change in a more sudden way. For example, a grandparent or other relative dies; you find out that you are moving to another city or country; or your parents are getting a divorce.

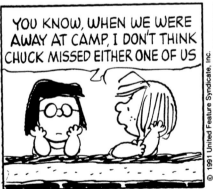
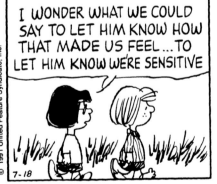
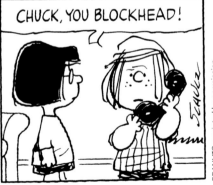

How might Patty's comment to Chuck create stress in their friendship? What could Patty have said instead?

Signs of Stress

We all react differently to stress. Some people might feel tired all the time but aren't able to sleep. Others might eat too much or not feel like eating at all. Still others might not be able to concentrate. Stress can make you feel sad, or angry, or crabby. It could put you in a bad mood for no reason. Sometimes stress can give you a headache or make you feel sick to your stomach. In other words, you don't feel like yourself when you feel stressed.

When someone has experienced an especially difficult change or loss, the signs of stress can become more serious. These are some of the symptoms:

- pretending that nothing has happened because you don't want to believe that something did happen

- withdrawing from friends

- feeling angry at the situation or the person who is causing the hurt

- blaming yourself for what happened

In some cases, parts of your life will be different as a result of this change or loss, so give yourself time to recover.

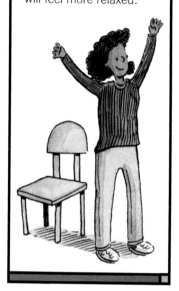

PHYSICAL ACTIVITY TODAY

Stress can make your muscles tense. When you feel stressed, take five minutes to stretch. You will feel more relaxed.

MOVING? THINK POSITIVELY!

Moving can be a difficult period for everyone because it can mean leaving friends, family, and familiar places. It can also be exciting because it means new friends, a new school, and a new neighbourhood. If you are feeling stressed about your move, talk to your family about how you feel. Get to know your new community. Check it out on the Internet. Think positively about this change in your life. Once you move, join activities at school and in your community. You'll meet people with similar interests to yours. And keep in touch with your old friends through mail, phone, or e-mail.

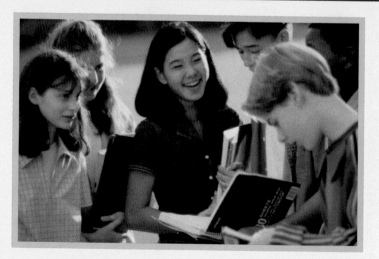

Get your friends' postal and e-mail addresses so you can keep in touch with them after you've moved.

How to Help Yourself

Stress may be a normal part of relationships, but it still isn't much fun. You can deal with stress in healthy ways. The first step in dealing with stress is to know that you *can* do something about it.

Here's what you can do:

- Talk with a friend. You might find that your friend has the same problems.

- Talk with a parent, or another adult you trust.

- Accept support from your friends when they offer it.

- Keep connected with people in your life who care about you.

- Accept that there are some things you cannot change or control, and then focus on what you can change.

- Remember that feelings of stress can grow if the issue is not dealt with in some way.

If you need help with your problems, you may want to get help from someone who is trained to deal with stress. Talking with a school counsellor, community health worker, doctor, social worker, psychologist, or grief counsellor can help you deal with long-term stress.

Here's a Hint

Getting help for an emotional problem is the same as getting help for any other problem. It doesn't mean you're "crazy." It means that you are mature enough to look for ways to solve your problems instead of letting them become worse. Getting the right kind of help can make you feel a lot better.

Talking with an adult you trust can help you cope with stress. Adults can help you see the problem from a different perspective because they may have been through similar problems themselves.

You Can Help Too

You might not be the one with the problem. If your friends are upset, you can support them by listening to their problems and trying to understand what they are going through. Sometimes inviting them to do something with you can help. Don't force them, but let them know you care and want to be with them. If you can't help with the problem, encourage them to talk to someone who can help. Offer to go with them to talk to an adult they can trust.

Here's a Hint

When you listen to a friend talk about a problem, try not to say, "I know what you mean," and then go on to talk about yourself or a problem you have. There are times when you need to be the listener.

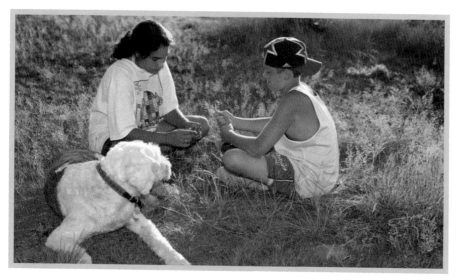

Talking to a friend about your problem can help you work out a solution.

Over to You

1. a) **Just for You:** Think of the last time you felt stress because something was happening with a friend. What was the event? What did you do?

   b) Would you do the same thing now? What would you change?

2. With a partner, brainstorm a list of five situations in which teens might need emotional support. What is one way you could help in each situation? Take turns role-playing these situations.

3. As a class, make a list of health or other community resources within your town or city where teens can get help with issues such as depression, dealing with loss and grief, and other topics that might cause teens stress.

4. **Just for You:** Make a list of the people you could turn to for emotional support.

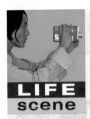

LIFE scene

Helping Friends Cope

Read the following scenarios and think about how you would help your friend in each situation.

Dana

seems really depressed. She doesn't want to go out. She's not doing her homework. Dana says she feels terrible but that she can't help the way she feels. She appears to have the perfect life—with a good family and great friends.

Ravi

thinks he's being picked on by his French teacher. He says he's *always* singled out for blame when the entire class is talking. Ravi has tried talking to the teacher about it, but the teacher just keeps telling him it's his fault.

Fadia

is very upset. Her grandmother died three months ago. Fadia says she misses her so much and that she cries herself to sleep almost every night. She can't concentrate and her school work is suffering. Fadia is avoiding her friends and doesn't talk to them on the phone.

Anthony

is going through a hard time at home. His parents recently went through a divorce. His mother had to get a job. As a result, Anthony has to go home every day right after school to pick up his little brother from kindergarten. He can't make practices any more. He's tried to talk to his mom about it, but she says he'll just have to get used to it.

Amy

lives with a parent who is an alcoholic. When her father drinks, her mother gets angry and there is always yelling and arguing— sometimes through the entire night. This fighting has been going on for more than a year now. Amy said she just wants to run away from it all.

◀◀ Now You Know

→ Thoughts and emotions are linked; they influence each other.

→ You can change a negative thinking pattern into a positive one through positive self-talk and visualizations.

→ Relationships have times of stress. There are many ways to deal with this stress and other stresses in your life.

→ Even if you just listen to someone who has a problem, you are being a great help to that person.

→ Your friends, parents, and other adults, including school counsellors and health care professionals, are all sources of support.

↻ Over to You

1. How would positive thinking help you in the following situations?

a) You do well in your public speaking presentation, but you don't come in first.

b) You have an argument with your parents and now you are grounded for the weekend.

c) You can't go to a movie with friends because you have to babysit your younger sister.

2. In your notebook, make a table like the one below.

Fill in the columns using the following situations:

a) not doing very well on my science unit test

b) missing my serve for the fourth time in a volleyball game

c) having an argument with my best friend

d) forgetting to do my book report for English class

e) learning that my family is moving to another city

f) learning that my pet has died

Problem or Situation	Explanation to Myself	My Feelings

Key terms

feedback,
win/lose,
lose/lose,
win/win

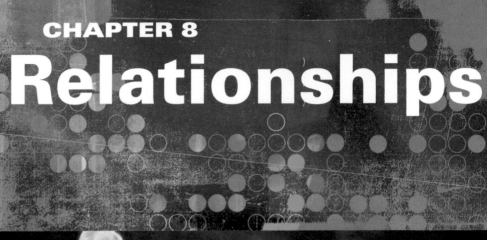

CHAPTER 8
Relationships

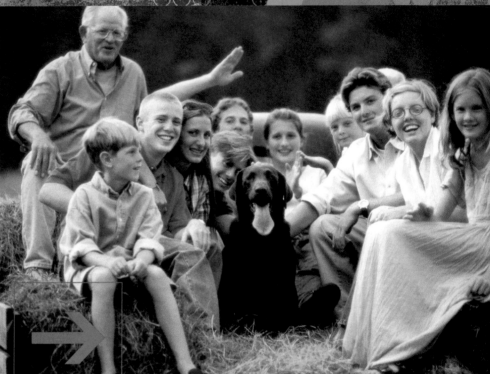

Let's Go!

Imagine a world where choosing a new best friend is done with an interview.

→ Write three questions that you would ask someone to find out whether that person would be a good friend.

→ Do you think it is possible to describe a friendship? Why or why not?

Relationships in Life

Relationships come in all shapes and sizes. Some are new; some have been with us since we were born. Relationships can happen anywhere. In this chapter, you will learn about the qualities that make healthy relationships. You will examine ways to resolve conflicts in a relationship. You will also see how media violence may influence the way some people handle conflict.

What Are Relationships?

Relationships are connections with others. Relationships grow and change. With care, they can become better. They can also end.

To keep a relationship strong, both people need to give to it. This does not mean giving presents. It means giving support, friendship, time, and respect. Just as each person gives, each person receives. The "give and receive" is an ongoing part of every healthy relationship.

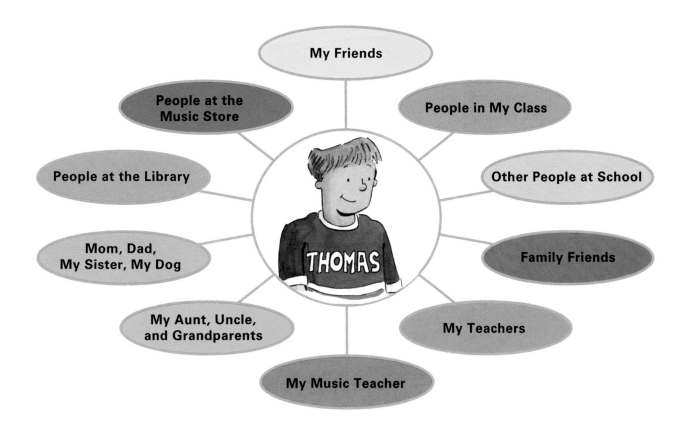

Healthy Relationships

What is a healthy relationship? It is a partnership that is enjoyed by both people who want to be in the relationship. A healthy relationship has certain qualities. People in a healthy relationship make an effort to:

❋ have good **communication.** Communication involves talking and listening. It means sharing your thoughts, feelings, and opinions. It also means accepting the thoughts, feelings, and opinions of the other person. People in a relationship may not always agree, but they respect each other.

❋ feel **comfortable** sharing information. Neither of you should feel embarrassed about what you say. You should not worry that the other person will put you down.

❋ **understand** each other. To know someone, you have to try to understand as much as you can about that person. You should know about each other's likes, dislikes, interests, and concerns. But you do not have to share the same opinions to have a good relationship.

❋ **care** about each other. You know what cheers up the other person. You also know what might hurt that person. Caring also involves loyalty and trust. Being loyal to a friend includes not gossiping about that person. It also means not sharing that person's personal information with others.

❋ **co-operate** with each other. A relationship is based on giving, receiving, and sharing. This means that there has to be co-operation between the two people.

❋ **appreciate** each other. Both people in a relationship need to know that they are valued. They need to know that they are important to each other.

Relationships Need Feedback

Zach slaps the puck into the net.

Yari yells, "Good shot."

Zach smiles and nods at Yari as he skates away.

Communication is about sending and receiving messages. When Zach makes a great shot, Yari sends a "good job" message to him. Zach receives that message and lets Yari know it was received by smiling and nodding. Yari and Zach are communicating with each other by sending messages and giving **feedback** to each other.

Feedback is a response to a message that has been sent. It lets the sender know that the message was received and that it was understood. It gives a reaction to the message. Positive feedback can be a wave, a smile, or a thumbs-up. Or it can be a short statement letting someone know he or she is liked, appreciated, or has done a good job. It is also a way of showing that someone's opinion is valued. A compliment can be positive feedback. Positive feedback can make people feel good.

Negative feedback can make people feel bad. It can say things such as your thoughts are not welcome, you are not valued, or I don't like you.

feedback: response to another person's message

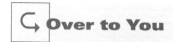

Over to You

Give yourself some positive feedback. Write yourself a positive message and put it in your pocket, then read it later in the day.

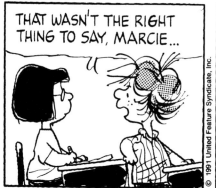
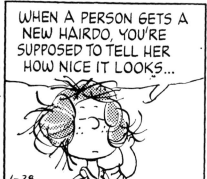
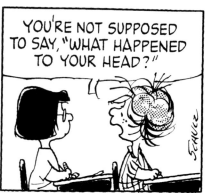

Why is positive feedback important?

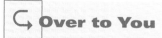

Over to You

With a partner, brainstorm two examples of positive feedback that someone could give to a person at school, at home, and to a friend. Make your examples as realistic as possible. Role-play these situations to practise giving and receiving feedback.

Friends

Here's a Hint

Friends can make mistakes. Sometimes friends might hurt your feelings, but friendships require forgiveness and acceptance.

A friend is someone you choose and who chooses you. Usually this person is not a relative. A friend is a choice. Friends like each other's company and freely agree to be together. Friends can be male or female; they can be younger or older than you.

Friendships are not perfect, just as the people who make up the friendships are not perfect. A friend might tease you or be inconsiderate, but these times should be rare. A good friendship has some bad times, but it also has many good times.

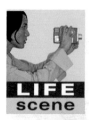

LIFE scene

Friendships

Think about the qualities that make a relationship healthy. Describe the qualities of friendship found in the examples below. Explain how these qualities help each friendship.

Eric and Mr. Whitten

are neighbours. Every day, on his way home from school, Eric stops by Mr. Whitten's house. Mr. Whitten is retired and enjoys Eric's visits. Eric always looks forward to discussing his day with Mr. Whitten. Sometimes the two of them work on the model train system in the living room.

Patricia and Scott

enjoy each other's company and spend a good deal of time together. They are not "boyfriend/girlfriend." They are simply good friends. In the summer, they go cycling together, and in the winter, they ski together. Sometimes they go to the movies with a group of friends. Patricia and Scott really enjoy talking and joking with each other.

Vinay and Alex

walk home from school together every day. On the way home, they always talk. Vinay has difficulty with math problems while Alex finds them easy. Alex helps Vinay with math. Last summer Vinay taught Alex to swim. Then both boys took a swimming test and passed. They decided to celebrate by going to a movie.

Changing Relationships

Sometimes friends do not see each other for a long time, yet their friendship remains strong. Not all friendships can survive long breaks though. Friends may drift apart for many reasons. Read the following scenario and think about why some friendships change.

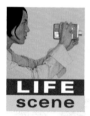

LIFE scene

Together or Apart?

Alan and Brad had a great time at camp last summer. They were in the same group every day and spent almost all their time together. When camp ended, they were both disappointed that they would not see each other for a long time, perhaps not even until next summer at camp.

Alan and Brad had a chance to see each other over the winter break. They got to see each other almost every day.

What do you think happened?

Together

Alan and Brad had a great week. It was like they had never been apart. They went to movies, played computer games, went skating, and talked into the late hours of the night. When the week ended, both Alan and Brad knew that they would get to see each other again. And they knew they had a good friendship.

Apart

Alan and Brad were happy to see each other. They hung out together on the first day but didn't seem to have much to talk about. They went to a movie but had a difficult time agreeing on which one to see. One night they went skating. Alan spent most of the time talking to other kids, and Brad spent most of the time skating alone. By the end of the week, they hadn't seen each other for a couple of days. In fact, both Alan and Brad were having a good time doing other things.

Explain how Alan and Brad's friendship has changed in each situation. Why is it a good thing that some friendships change?

Making It Better

Sometimes we take good relationships for granted. We assume that our relationships will last without any effort on our part. That is not always the case. Think about what it would be like to never get anything from a friend—no attention, no positive feedback, no time together. Eventually, how do you think you would feel?

If something is going wrong in a relationship, try to find out what is going wrong and why. Don't avoid your friend. Instead find a quiet moment and ask what has happened. Be sure to really listen to the answer, if there is one.

⤷ Over to You

Think about friendships you had in the past. Why do you think that these friendships ended?

VIP! VERY IMPORTANT POINT

Some relationships cannot be fixed. A relationship can be fixed only if both people want to fix it. If one person wants to end a relationship, the other person has to let that happen.

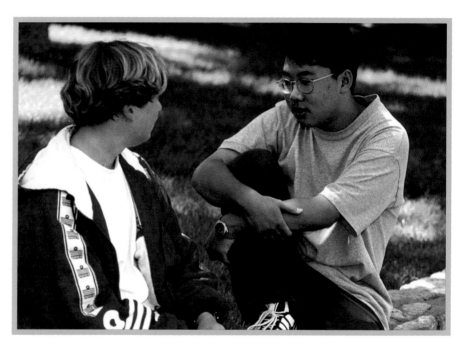

Relationships take work. Sometimes you talk, and sometimes you listen.

⤷ Over to You

1. Create an illustration to show the relationships that are close to you.

2. Create a poster or write a poem that explains why friendship is important.

3. Describe two simple things a person can do to show that he or she cares for a family member.

4. Describe a situation when it might be better to end a relationship than to try to make it better.

Conflict in Relationships

All relationships have ups and downs and disagreements. Each person in a relationship has ideas and opinions. Sometimes people disagree and there is conflict. Call them arguments, quarrels, or squabbles. When there are times of conflict, there are ways to deal with it.

If something is wrong in a relationship, you need to take the following actions if you want to make it better.

* **Step one:** Find out what is wrong. Maybe it is just a misunderstanding, and simply understanding the situation can solve the problem.

* **Step two:** Talk about the problem. What does each person want? Is there a way both of you can have what you want? If so, then agree to it.

* **Step three:** If there is no way you can both have what you want, find the best solution for each of you. Is there a possibility that you can take turns getting what you want? Is it OK for each of you to get some of what you want?

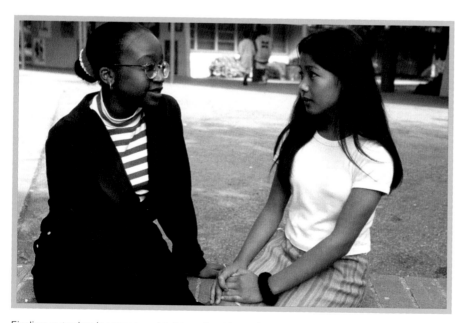

Finding out what is wrong and talking about it are important steps in resolving conflict.

How to Talk About a Problem

Talking about your problem is not always easy to do. Start by expressing your opinions and thoughts clearly. Don't exaggerate the problem. And listen to the opinions and thoughts of the other person. Here are some other tips:

* Remain calm. Insults and rudeness will offend the other person, and he or she will stop listening to what you are saying.

* Control your temper. Losing your "cool" will only make the situation worse.

* Do not sulk, pout, or withdraw. These actions will keep you from reaching a good solution.

* Remember: A disagreement does not mean that people like each other less.

It is important for both people to feel as though they have been treated fairly.

Finding the Best Solution

Have you ever had an argument that left both you and the other person angry? You probably thought there should have been a better solution. If one person leaves the discussion feeling displeased, then there *was* a better way to deal with the problem. Take a look at the following ways of handling a disagreement.

Win/Lose: One person is happy, one person is not.

Many people think that if someone wins, the other person has to lose. That is why they choose a **win/lose** solution. The truth is both people lose something with this kind of solution. The winner can lose a good friendship. Even small arguments are damaging to a relationship, because each time someone loses, the relationship shrinks a little.

Here's a Hint

If your solution is always win/lose, that means you are going to be the loser some of the time. Is this what you want?

Lose/Lose: Both people are unhappy.

A **lose/lose** solution is the worst choice people can make. No one wins. It is almost as if the people involved feel the solution is fair because both are unhappy. It is a terrible choice—there must be a better way!

Win/Win: Both people are pleased.

Choosing a **win/win** solution requires working together to figure out the best choice. Sometimes it is as simple as talking about the problem and then agreeing on a solution. If you both feel happy with the solution, then you have both won.

But sometimes coming up with a win/win solution takes even more thinking than the argument itself. Figure out the best options together. Each person should get a solution that is acceptable, even pleasing. Take pride in the fact that you think the relationship is important enough to be worth the work. Think of the problem as a puzzle and solve it together.

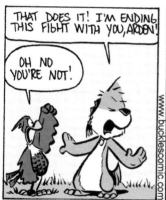 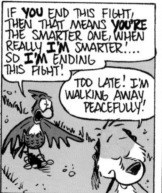 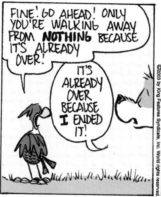 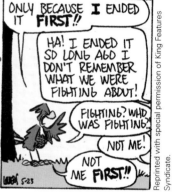

How is this disagreement being handled? How will it work out?

Improving Relationships

Perfect relationships do not exist. But you can improve your relationships with family, friends, classmates, and others by treating people well. You will be surprised at people's reactions the first few times you say something nice or do something extra for them.

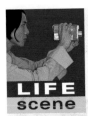

LIFE scene

Finding a Solution

Using what you know about working together, suggest some actions the families below could take to reach a win/win solution for their disagreements.

Dari

needs some new clothes. She wants a pair of shoes like the ones that her friend just bought. Dari's mom says "no." Dari is furious. She even offers to do more work around the house, but the answer is still "no."

Ed

thinks it is silly that he has to be home on weeknights long before his friends have to. He decides to stay out late one night. When he gets home that night, his parents are upset.

Neil

likes to spend a couple of hours a day playing video games at the neighbourhood store. He uses the money that he has earned delivering flyers. Last night his dad told him he couldn't hang around the store any more.

↪ Over to You

1. As a class, brainstorm examples of conflict in relationships. Include examples of conflict at school, at home, with friends, and with classmates. Then work in small groups to find good solutions to some of these conflicts. As a class, discuss the different solutions.

2. With a partner, role-play a win/win solution to one of the conflicts presented in the above Life Scene.

Relationships and Media Violence

Have you ever known a child who watches cartoons of animals involved in kick-boxing and then starts kicking people when she doesn't get her own way? Why do you think this happens?

The violence you see in the media is often more dangerous than a child trying to kick-box. How about a movie where one person slaps another person during an argument? Or a video where someone is beaten to solve a problem? Or a computer game where bodies have to be blown apart in order to win? Because we know that these scenes are fiction, we might think that we are not influenced by the violence in them. But many experts feel that violence in the media can influence people's behaviour. They believe it can influence how people treat each other.

We need to be concerned about the power of seeing violence in movies, videos, computer games, and on TV. Such images can lead us to believe that problems in real life can be solved through violence. Violent images can also convince people that it is OK to use violence to get what they want. Violence in relationships is never acceptable. Violence is always harmful to a relationship.

VIP! VERY IMPORTANT POINT

Some people believe that seeing violence in the media makes us less sensitive to real acts of violence. They believe this makes us more accepting of violence in the real world.

↪ Over to You

1. Create an action plan for dealing with the violence you see in the media.

a) Start by thinking about where you see media violence. Do you see it on TV? Do you see it in computer games?

b) Think about what you will do the next time you see violence in the media. (Hint: Remind yourself that the violence in movies, videos, and computer games is invented. Think about non-violent ways the same situations could have been handled.)

c) Now decide what actions you can take to reduce the amount of media violence that you see.

d) What can you do for other people, especially children, when it comes to watching media violence?

◀◀ Now You Know

→ A healthy relationship relies on certain qualities—communication, feeling comfortable, understanding, caring, co-operation, and appreciation.

→ Feedback is an important part of the communication process.

→ The strength of a friendship depends on the people involved and their willingness to work on building the relationship.

→ There are various styles of conflict resolution—win/lose, lose/lose, and win/win.

→ Talking about a problem and listening to the opinions and thoughts of the other person can resolve disagreements. A fair solution can be reached by talking and listening.

→ Displays of violence in the media can lead to violent behaviour in relationships.

↳ Over to You

1. a) Have you ever been part of an unhealthy friendship?

   b) How did you know that the friendship was unhealthy?

   c) Write about your experience.

2. Have you ever ignored someone who was talking to you? Have you ever been ignored? What does this do to communication? Suggest ways to fix the situation.

3. a) As a class, brainstorm a list of specific examples of violent scenes on television, in books, in movies, in music videos, and in computer and video games.

   b) In small groups, choose three examples from the list. For each example, answer the following questions:

   i) Why is the violence used?

   ii) What happened after the violence?

   iii) How might people react to the same situation in real life?

   c) Suggest non-violent ways to resolve the issues that you came up with in part (a).

Working Together

Key terms

group, team,
collaboration,
gang, initiation,
conform

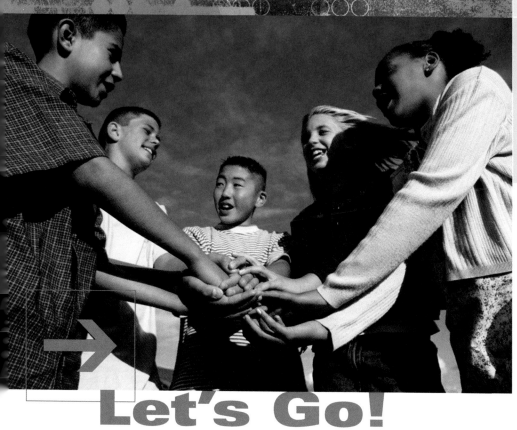

Let's Go!

→ Name a group that you think works well together. It could be a group on TV, in a movie, or a real group you know.

→ Describe one decision this group has made.

→ Did this decision work for the group? Why or why not?

Groups

There are many words used to describe groups. Wolves hunt in packs, whales travel in pods, and fish swim in schools. Groups of people may be called cliques, clubs, and crews, just to name a few. Groups are all around us. Imagine that you are standing on the second floor of a shopping mall, looking at the people below. When you look closely into the crowd, you can see small groups—families, young children chasing each other, and teens laughing and walking together.

In this chapter, you will examine the differences among groups, teams, and gangs. You will also see how to be a member of a winning team and how to make a difference in your community.

What Is a Group?

group: a collection of people who share something in common

A **group** is more than just a collection of people. Group members have something in common, such as similar interests or goals. Whether you are with friends, on a sports team, in a club, or part of a project at school, you are a member of a group.

Groups are a natural part of life. Some groups, such as a circle of friends, form naturally. Other groups, such as sports teams and student work groups, are created for a purpose.

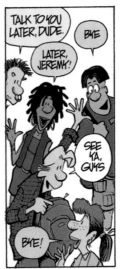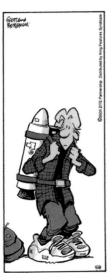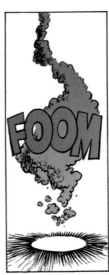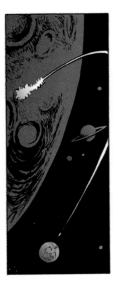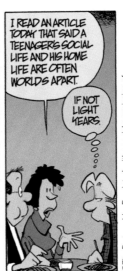

The interests you share with one group may be quite different from the interests you share with another group.

Choosing Groups

There are important reasons to think about the groups you choose to join. A group can influence how you act and how you think about things. Being in a group tells the world a lot about you. Your choice of groups now will also influence your future. What you learn and how you act in a group now will always be part of you. There may be times when you find out that a group you wanted to be part of is not what you thought it was. Because you are an individual, you can choose not to be a group member. You can change your mind.

There are certain benefits to belonging to a group. Of course, the benefits will vary depending on the type of group.

Here's a Hint

Remember: Much of what you do reflects the people you choose to spend time with and what they choose to do.

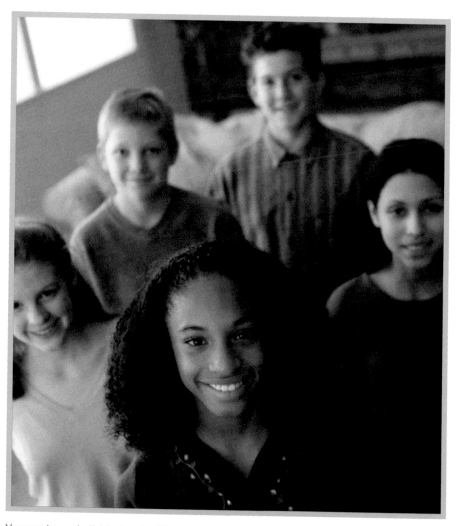

You can be an individual and still be part of a group. As a group member, you can do what you think is right, even when other members don't agree with you.

* You can spend time with people who share your interests. You can feel as if you belong.

* You can be liked for who you are and what you do. You can feel confident about yourself.

* You can get to know yourself better. Talking with others can help you to understand what you think and why you think that way. You can choose how you show yourself to others.

* You can learn new skills, including how to act in new situations and how to handle new relationships. With new skills, you can feel more independent and you can be proud of new accomplishments.

* You can get support and assistance when you need it. You can also give support to others when they need it.

* You can have fun! A lot of things are more fun to do with other people than by yourself. Going places, playing games, and laughing are a lot more fun with a group of friends.

Here's a Hint

When you talk with other people, you *hear* what you are thinking. Belonging to a group gives you the chance to share your thoughts and ideas with others.

Danger! Pressure

You need to pay attention any time you are feeling pressured by a group. Little alarms should go off in your head.

You need to take action if you are being pressured to:

* do something that doesn't feel right or that you know is wrong, especially if it is something that is illegal

* treat another person badly, including making fun of someone, embarrassing someone, or worse

* spend less time with other friends or your family

You know when you are being pressured. You may feel uncomfortable about doing something. Or you may do something you don't want to in order to be accepted by the group. It can be hard to take a stand in a group. But being part of a group does not take away your brain. In fact, if you aren't allowed to think for yourself, then it's not the group for you.

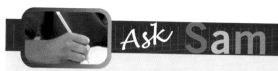

Dear Sam,

I like my bunch of friends. We usually do crazy stuff and have a good time.

The problem is that the newest thing is to shoplift. We have never done anything like this before. I don't want to do it, but my friends are making fun of me. They say that stores expect people to shoplift, so I shouldn't worry. One guy said I was "chicken." I don't know what to do.

Help!

Pressured

Dear Pressured,

Not wanting to do something illegal is not being chicken, it's being smart. Here are some things you should do:

- Ask yourself what would really happen if you chose not to do it. Not every choice you make will get you kicked out of the group. A lot of groups have members who do different things.

- Speak out. Express your point of view. Members of a group should have the right to talk.

- Don't do it. And don't tag along. If you're hanging with shoplifters, it will be tough to convince people that you aren't shoplifting too. The best motto: Do only what you feel right about doing.

Sam

⌐ Over to You

1. Have you ever heard about a group of teens being asked to leave a convenience store because there were "too many of them" in the store?

   a) Why do you think this happens?

   b) Describe a situation when you were treated unfairly because you were with a group of teens.

2. Working on your own, write about a group that has been important to you. It might be a circle of friends, a group of relatives, a club, or some other group. Describe the group and explain why it has been important.

Teams

What makes a group of people a team? We commonly think of a **team** in terms of sports, but any group of people who work together to achieve a common goal is a team. The goal might be raising money for a school field trip, winning a soccer game, or working on a school project. A group with a goal can get a lot done. This will only happen if the members know the goal, can work well together, and have a plan to achieve the goal. Working *as a team* is how a group gets things done.

team: a group of people working together toward a common goal

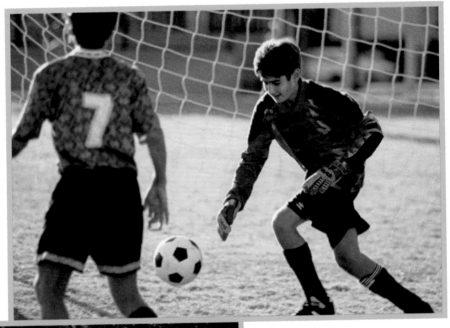

Playing well together to win a game or working together to raise money for a cause are examples of common goals that a team might have.

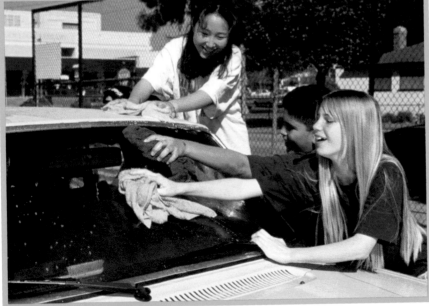

Building a Winning Team

A team is successful when its members figure out how to work well together. Working well together is called **collaboration.** Here are ways a successful team collaborates:

collaboration: working well together to achieve a goal

The team has good communication.

- Members talk with one another and discuss topics.

- The discussions are not arguments.

- Members listen to one another.

- Each member has a chance to talk.

⤾ **Over to You**

Brainstorm a list of groups that work together as a team. Then identify the goals that each group might have.

Each member works to carry out the plan.

- Each member is responsible for his or her own job and doesn't allow others to do all the work.

- Members have to work together to make the plan work.

Members respect themselves and the others on the team.

- Members do their own jobs. They do not do another member's job, but they do help one another.

- Members respect the leader and work with that person.

- The leader sees the value of each member. The leader respects each member.

- Members work to get along with one another.

The team gets stronger as it works together.

- Members get better at making decisions and solving problems together.

- Members are proud of their work.

Working Together Toward a Goal

Why are goals so important? Because they move you from "here" to "where you want to be." Having a goal is what moves you forward. This is true for individuals and for groups. Without a goal, a group may want to do something but may never be able to get there. The members may do a lot of work, but the group doesn't really accomplish anything. A group has to know and agree on a goal. Any group that knows its goal can work toward success.

Whether you are a group of friends who have chosen your own goal or a group of students who have been given a class assignment, you can work toward a common goal. Here's how:

1. Decide on a goal and agree to work together. Be sure to write out the goal so that everyone can see it.

2. Make an action plan. List the steps to reach your goal. Then list the tasks that need to be done. Make another list of the resources you will need. Set some deadlines.

3. Figure out what each member must do to make the group successful. Beside each task on the lists, write the name of the member responsible for that task. Make sure that all members understand their responsibilities.

4. Each member now begins work. Meet once in a while to review the goal and check on each person's progress. Help one another when needed.

5. Celebrate the team's success. Praise one another.

⤷ Over to You

1. In this activity, you will be working in groups to achieve a goal. Your task is to choose one important health message and communicate it to other students in your school.

   a) As a group, brainstorm a list of positive ideas about health. Then choose one important idea.

   b) Choose a way to communicate this message. For example, create posters and flyers, add the message to the school Web site, or do a skit.

   c) Follow the steps listed in Working Together Toward a Goal. Describe what your group will do for each step.

   d) Present your completed plan to the class.

2. As a class, choose one or more of these plans and use it to spread a positive health message to other students. Celebrate your success.

Gangs

Gangs are usually identified as groups of people who are involved in illegal and sometimes violent activities. These activities include shoplifting, vandalism, and theft. Gangs are a concern in some Canadian communities and schools.

Gangs are like other groups in some ways. Members of gangs are usually interested in the same things, and they get support from one another. But the main difference between gangs and other kinds of groups is that gangs do things that are illegal.

In a gang, there is a leader who establishes the "laws" for other members. Becoming a member is an important act. There may be an **initiation,** which is a joining ceremony. Members have to promise to be loyal. They may have to prove their loyalty. If they are not loyal, they can be punished.

Members identify one another and show loyalty to the gang by what they wear. They may wear certain colours, clothes, or jewellery. They may have tattoos or body piercings. Wearing the same clothes or having the same tattoos makes members feel like part of a group.

Gang members are accepted only if they **conform.** They have to act in ways the leader and other members demand. Once someone becomes a member, leaving the gang can be difficult. It can be dangerous to leave or even talk about leaving.

gang: a group of people united by illegal activity and acts of violence

initiation: a test someone takes to show loyalty and obedience

conform: to accept and follow the rules

↪ Over to You

As a class, discuss the following questions:

• Are gangs a concern in your school?

• What do you think schools should do about gangs?

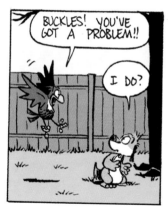
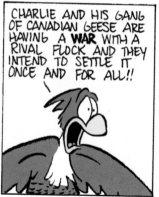
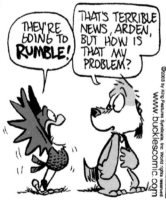
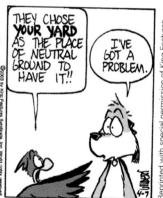
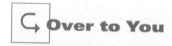

Rival gangs often fight for control over territory.

Why Do People Join Gangs?

People join gangs for a variety of reasons. Some young people join gangs because they don't feel supported by family and friends. Being a member of a gang makes them feel as though they belong somewhere. Being part of a gang may also give them a recognition they aren't getting at home. Other people join gangs in order to:

- have a reputation for being in a gang, which makes them feel important

- feel accepted

- be protected and have the support of other gang members

- stop the harassment and pressure from gang members to join them

- be safe, and sometimes even to stay alive

Some people may join a gang because they believe being part of a gang is the only way they can develop a close relationship with others. However, some studies show that even though gang members spend a lot of time together, they seldom describe their relationships with fellow members as being close.

↪ Over to You

1. You have just read a section called "Why Do People Join Gangs?" Imagine that you are a textbook writer and write a section called "Reasons Not to Join a Gang."

2. The word used to describe a group can give you information about that group.

   a) What would you think if your teacher asked your class to divide into three gangs to do a class activity?

   b) Would it be different if your teacher asked your class to divide into three groups? If so, how?

   c) Would it be different if your teacher asked your class to divide into three teams? Explain the difference.

   d) Which word do you like best? Why?

3. Find out what your city, town, or community is doing about gangs. Suggest other things that could be done about this problem.

QuickQuiz

Group, Team, or Gang?

Make a table in your notebook with the following headings:

Group   Team   Gang

Indicate by number which of the following statements describe a group, a team, or a gang. Statements can be used more than once.

1. Members spend time with people who want to be together.

2. Members work to develop and improve skills.

3. Members are free to leave any time.

4. Getting together is organized and scheduled.

5. Members can be pressured to do things that are wrong.

6. Members have a set goal or purpose and work together to achieve it.

7. Each member can choose how to act.

8. Members embarrass or hurt people who are not included.

9. Each member is important and needed.

10. A person has to work hard to be allowed to join the group.

11. Members have to do a lot of things to be accepted by the group.

12. The group does unlawful activities.

13. Membership is kept secret from outsiders.

14. Members have fun together.

15. People feel proud to be members.

16. Members are not allowed to spend time with old friends or groups.

17. Members don't have a lot of problems or hassles with one another.

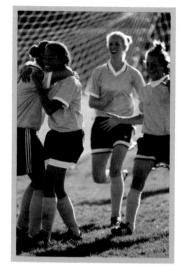

Positive feedback is important in teamwork. Positive feedback means letting others know when they have done a good job.

⤷ Over to You

As you probably learned from the Quick Quiz, some of the same statements could be used to describe groups, teams, and gangs. That makes sense because groups, teams, and gangs all have some things in common. But they also have things that make them different.

Review the 17 statements in the Quick Quiz and choose 5 that *best* describe the characteristics of a team. Do the same for a group and for a gang. Then write your own descriptions for a group, a team, and a gang.

Making a Difference in Your Community

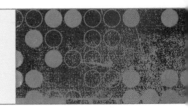

The health of your community depends on the care and attention it gets from the people who live there. Individuals and groups can contribute to a safe and caring environment.

Now that you have learned about working in a group, you can use this information to set and achieve a group goal. As a class, choose a project that will improve the health of your school, neighbourhood, or community. Below is a list of some ways you can become involved in order to make a difference in your community.

- Study your school or neighbourhood and prepare an inventory of possible health concerns. Suggest steps that caring groups can take to address these concerns.

- Plan a recycling project. Identify materials that you would need and methods that you could use to recycle products. Suggest ways you can convince others to adopt your plan.

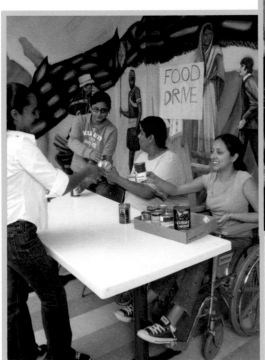

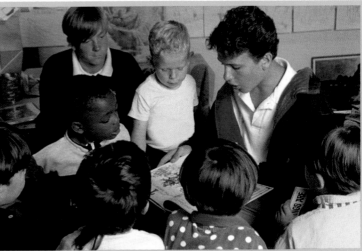

Working at a food drive or reading to children are two ways of helping others in your community.

- Organize a spring cleanup team in your neighbourhood. Include a map of the area and list tasks for each team member. Suggest ways to convince others in the community to participate.

- Create posters with positive messages about health. Post them in the classroom, the school, and the community.

- Plan to plant trees on the school grounds or in a playground close to you. Find out how you can get the proper permission to do this. Use your school newsletter or community newspaper to let the community know about your plans and to invite donations and assistance.

- Contact your local Society for the Prevention of Cruelty to Animals (SPCA) and ask what supplies they need for animal care. Create a flyer that describes your project and lists the needed supplies. Then ask the people in your neighbourhood if they would like to donate any of the supplies.

- Check out some optometrists, stores that sell eyeglasses, and the local Canadian National Institute for the Blind (CNIB) to learn about any programs that send used eyeglasses to people in need. Gather old eyeglasses and donate them to a program.

- Investigate how you can help other people in your community through a food bank or local kitchen. Then help out by donating your time or by raising money.

- Volunteer to read to children or adults in your community.

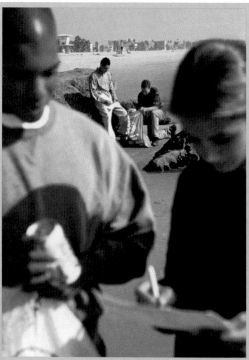

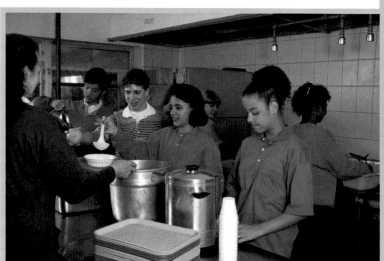

Volunteering in a soup kitchen or participating in a project to improve the environment are two other ways of helping out in your community.

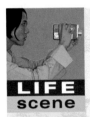

The Tree Team

It all started when vandals set fire to the small treed park near the school. It was a popular park for many people, but for a group of five friends, it was an important part of every school day. This was the corner where they met on their way to school. They had been doing it for the last two years. Now the town had closed off the area.

At first, the five were angry. They were angry because the park was closed and because it was burned for no reason. They were also frustrated. It looked as though no one was going to clean up the area and make it safe.

Then one morning on the way to school, one member of the group suggested that they should get their own trees and plant them. Another member wondered how much trees would cost, and that got the conversation going. From there, they talked about the project. By the time they were at school, the group had a goal and a plan.

They knew that they didn't have enough money of their own and would need advice and help. They talked about it at school. A couple of other students offered to help. They talked about the plan with their families and some of their parents volunteered to help. By the weekend, the group was having its first car wash to help raise some money.

Over the next few weeks, the group raised more money and got the town's permission to clear the burned area. The local agri-culturalist provided advice. The local newspaper got interested in the group, and an article was written about them. A plant nursery donated pine seedlings and a few good-sized trees. There were more donations.

Over the next six months, the Tree Team (a dopey name the newspaper came up with) had become a group with 20 teens and many other volunteers. The group did a great job. Everyone had fun and felt good about accomplishing a project together.

◀◀ Now You Know

→ A group is a collection of people who interact regularly and share similar interests, values, or beliefs.

→ A group can influence how you act and think about things.

→ There are many advantages to belonging to a group.

→ A team is a group of people who work together to achieve a common goal.

→ A gang is a group of people united by violence and illegal activity.

→ Caring groups can change our world.

↻ Over to You

1. a) What was the goal of the Tree Team in the Life Scene on page 126?

b) What resources were used to reach the goal?

c) What were the obstacles that stood in the group's way?

d) If this group lived in your community, what projects could they do?

2. *Helping someone is good for your own health. Helping others can reduce feelings of stress and give you good feelings later when you remember what you did.*

As a class, discuss this statement. Give examples of how you have felt after helping others.

3. Working in small groups, consider the following project: Your group needs to raise $200 for an emergency fund to aid victims of a flood.

a) Decide what needs to happen in order to reach your goal.

b) Create a plan to reach your goal.

c) Discuss the tasks each person in your group could do.

d) Write out the steps your group would take to reach this goal.

e) Present your plan to the class.

Key terms

technology, portfolio, living document

CHAPTER 10

Thinking About Your Future

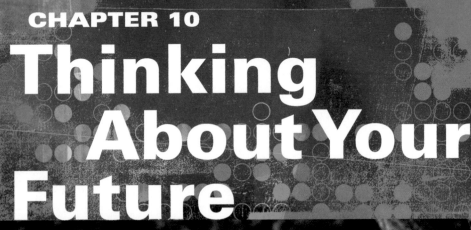

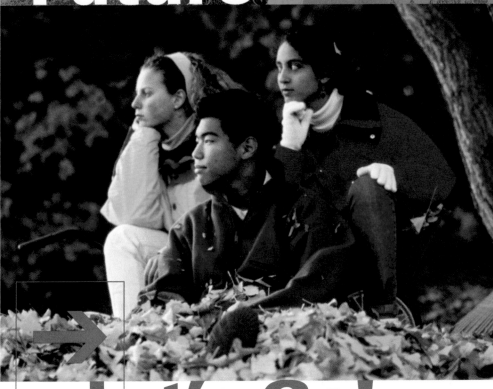

Let's Go!

→ Make a list of 10 discoveries and inventions that have changed our lives.

→ Choose the 2 that you think are the most important. Explain why you think each one is important to your life today.

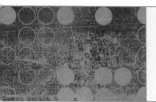

Why Think About the Future?

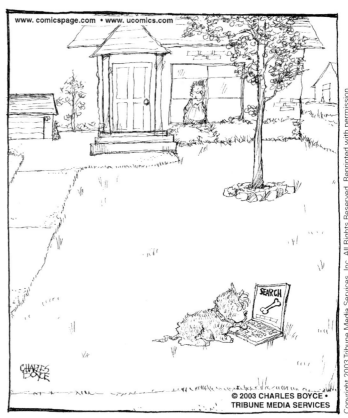

THANKS TO COMPUTER LESSONS IN OBEDIENCE SCHOOL, MURPHY HAS FEWER HOLES IN HIS YARD.

Many years ago, there were predictions that we would be jetting around in pods instead of driving cars. And robots would run our houses and do all the work!

We are still waiting for these predictions to come true. However, many discoveries and inventions have been made that no one could have ever imagined years ago. And new ones are appearing all the time.

By now you have learned how to set goals, make plans, and take action. You can use this information when you think about what you would like to see happen in the future. In this chapter, you will think about what you have to offer. You will consider some possibilities that interest you. You will also learn how to set long-term goals and how to create a personal portfolio.

Technology and Change

Technology is the use of new knowledge and scientific discoveries to create products and new ways of doing things. Technology helps us jump from "where we are now" to "into the future."

Technology changes lives. People have to adapt to the changes that technology brings. Jobs that require new types of education are created. Some jobs will no longer be needed.

When you think about your future, you should also think about technology. Think about the education you will need for new jobs. Think about the possibilities for your future.

technology: the use of new knowledge and discoveries to create new products and processes

1. **a)** Working in small groups, suggest some new discoveries, inventions, and ideas that would make big changes in:

- the world of sports
- how people travel
- how we could have peace in the world

b) Share your ideas with the class. Then post your ideas in the classroom.

QuickQuiz

Is This Real?

New technological advances can be surprising. Which of these discoveries and inventions are real and exist today? Which ones are dreams? Write the answers in your notebook. Then see page 141.

- A tiny crystal in the corner of one eyeglass lens is actually a computer monitor that allows you to read information about someone while talking face to face with that person.

- Treated sea coral is used as a bone graft to fix a badly broken leg.

- Communicate in any language by speaking into your hand-sized electronic translator. In a few seconds, your words will be spoken back to you in the language you select.

- If your cellphone battery runs down, look around for a public recharge booth. Just put in some coins, plug in your cellphone, and your phone will be recharged in just a few minutes.

- Send a video e-mail postcard to a friend from a phone and web-cam booth. Deposit money, make a quick video, and e-mail to a friend.

- Tired of holding the controller in your hands while playing a video game? Now you can use a dance pad. The control buttons on this floor mat are giant sized. You can stand up and stamp out your commands—and as a bonus, your body gets exercise while you play.

- A bandage with bacteria-sniffing microchips can detect specific germs (such as salmonella and E. coli) on your injured body. It then sends a message to a medical computer so that correct treatment can be started immediately.

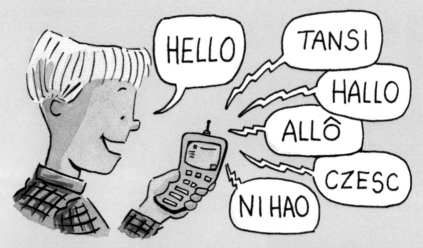

Translation: Tansi is Cree; Hallo is German; Allô is French; Czesc is Polish; and Ni hao is Mandarin.

Planning for Your Future

You can choose to plan for the future. In fact, if you plan, there are things you can do right now for the future. You can make choices about your future education and career possibilities. You can also make plans for far into the future.

Start Now!

Now it's time to gather data about you. This important information will be used later in the chapter when you create your personal portfolio.

1. Working in small groups, brainstorm all the possible suggestions to *one* of these topics:

   • things that interest us

   • skills and talents we have

   • our goals in life

   Make a list of all your suggestions on chart paper. Post all these lists around the classroom, grouping the same topics together. Save these charts of suggestions to use later in this chapter.

2. **Just for You:** Working on your own, create a personal list for *each* of the topics. These are now your private lists, and you do not have to share them with your classmates. For each topic, you should try to come up with 10 responses. Use the table below as a guide in making your lists. You can also use some of the ideas from your group list. Make sure you have at least 2 ideas of your own that are not part of the group list.

3. **Just for You:** Keep your lists nearby. You will need them later in this chapter.

Questions to Ask

Things That Interest Me	Skills and Talents I Have	My Goals in Life
• What do I enjoy doing?	• What do I do well?	• What careers interest me?
• What do I like to do...	• What skills do I have?	• Where do I want to work?
- outside?	• What are my talents?	• What type of work would I like to do?
- at home?	• What lessons and training do I have?	• What is the most important thing I want to do?
- with my friends?	• What competitions have I entered?	• And any other suggestions
- on my own?	• What are my volunteer experiences?	
- with my family?	• What types of work have I done?	
• What are my hobbies?	• And any other suggestions	
• What are my favourite things?		
• And any other suggestions		

Long-Term **Goals**

You already know that goals help to move you from "here" to "where you want to be." When it comes to long-term goals, the distance from "here" to "where you want to be" stretches fairly far into the future. More has to be done to reach a long-term goal than a short-term or medium-term goal. And you might face more challenges on the way to reaching your long-term goal.

The same process that helps you pin down your short-term and medium-term goals will be used to develop your long-term goals.

Goals   Set realistic goals that are possible to reach.

Obstacles   Recognize potential obstacles and work out solutions.

Action plan   Prepare a step-by-step plan to reach your goal.

Look, listen, learn   Use resources to find out what is required to achieve your goal.

Success   Identify what success will look like and measure your successes along the way.

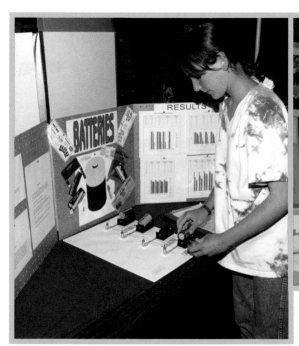
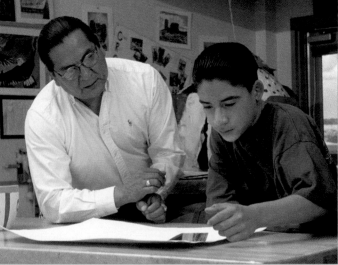

Reaching a long-term goal takes planning and work.

Is This Goal Realistic?

As you set a long-term goal, you need to think about whether it is realistic. Is it possible? Could it happen? Are you aware of things as they really are? Or is the goal so dream-like or imaginary that it could not possibly happen? Wanting to grow wings is not a realistic goal, but developing a new way to fly could be.

You need to consider your strengths, skills, and abilities. You need to make the best judgment you can. If it seems impossible to create an action plan, you might want to think about how realistic it is to reach the goal you have chosen.

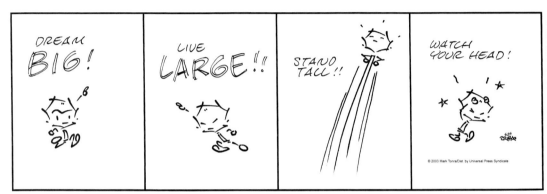

What do you think this cartoon strip is saying about goals?

Over to You

1. We can have many goals, different ones for different aspects of our lives. Think about the following areas of your life and suggest a goal for each.

   a) Personal – how you choose to live your life, how you choose to behave and show yourself to the world

   b) Social – your relationships with others, how you act and react with others

   c) Education – schooling now, types of education in the future, your responsibilities, your dreams

   d) Relaxation and Leisure – the ways you spend your time, your skills, your interests as they relate to leisure time

   e) Family – ways to enhance relationships

   f) Community – your neighbourhood, town, or city. What can you contribute?

Making CHOICES

Action Planning for the Future

Action planning for a long-term goal uses the process you already know, but there are a couple of changes. By asking the following questions, you can arrive at a plan for a long-term goal:

1. Where am I now?

2. Where do I want to be? What is my long-term goal? Is it realistic?

3. What actions or resources will get me there?

4. What is a realistic timeline for my action plan? For long-term goals, the timeline needs to be broken into several steps.

5. How am I doing along the way? At each step in the plan, review your progress and adjust the plan as needed.

6. How will I know whether I am successful?

The best thing about long-term goals and action planning for long-term goals is that you get to review your progress several times. You also have some time to adjust your plan before you actually reach your goal.

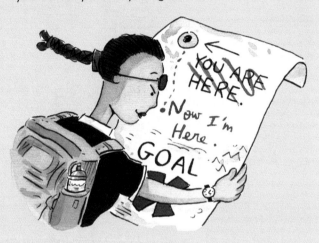

For long-term goals, check your progress often and adjust your plan so that you stay on target.

⤷ Over to You

1. Review the class lists of suggestions for Our Goals in Life (see page 131, question #1). Working in small groups, create an action plan for *one* of these suggested goals. Talk about each step in the action planning process. After you have discussed each step, record the group decision for that step. When complete, post your group's action plan in the classroom and explain it to the class.

2. Working on your own, create an action plan for *one* of the goals on your own list.

3. Write a paragraph to explain the importance of reviewing your progress and adjusting your plan from time to time.

Portfolios

rtists carry folders with samples of sketches and finished work. Sculptors carry albums of photographs. (It would be difficult to carry around large sculptures!) Architects carry blueprints and photographs of buildings in their briefcases. Actors show photographs, videos, newspaper articles, and reviews of their work to demonstrate what they have done. These people are using portfolios.

A **portfolio** is a collection of items organized for some purpose or goal. A portfolio may contain just a few items, or it may be quite large and have many items. However, you must remember that a portfolio is more than just a collection of things. What you choose to put in a portfolio and the way you organize those items must relate to your reason for having the portfolio.

A portfolio is one way to organize information about who you are and what you can do. It includes information about your interests, your skills, and some of your goals.

portfolio: a collection of items organized for a specific purpose

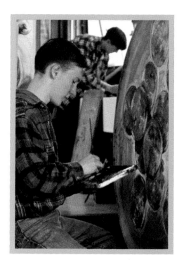

If a piece of art is too large for a portfolio, the artist can take a picture of the work and put it in the portfolio.

Building a Personal Portfolio

Portfolios come in all shapes, sizes, and forms. A portfolio can be a file folder, a three-ring binder, or even a shoebox. Some people create electronic portfolios on a floppy disk, on a CD, or even on a Web page. You will need to keep and use your personal portfolio over the next few years, so choose the format most convenient for you.

Portfolio Contents

Through the activities you have done, you have gathered information about your interests, your skills, and some of your goals. Your portfolio will feature this information.

Other items can be included in your portfolio. The next pages list just a few ideas. Choose items that you think are suitable for your portfolio. In some cases, a photocopy rather than the original item should be used. Turn the page to check out one student's portfolio.

My Portfolio

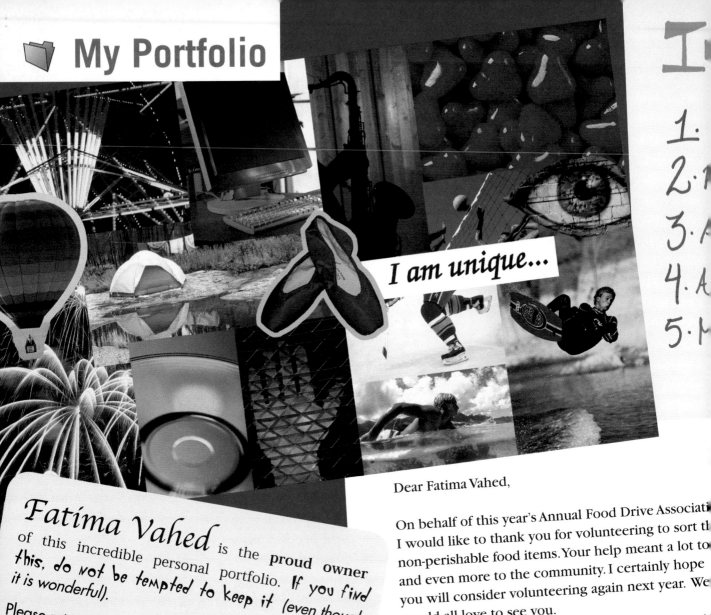

I am unique...

I

1.

2.

3.

4.

5.

Dear Fatima Vahed,

On behalf of this year's Annual Food Drive Associati
I would like to thank you for volunteering to sort th
non-perishable food items. Your help meant a lot to
and even more to the community. I certainly hope
you will consider volunteering again next year. We
would all love to see you.

Thank you once again. We couldn't have done i
without you.

Fatima Vahed is the **proud owner**
of this incredible personal portfolio. If you find
this, do not be tempted to keep it (even though
it is wonderful).

Please return to:
Parkside School, class 201.

Items for Portfolio

- A cover or first page that describes your interests or your goals.

- A return tag in case you lose your portfolio. Include your name, school name, and class number, or other information you think is important.

- A table of contents that lists all the pages and items in your portfolio. Remember that this portfolio will grow, so leave room for more entries.

- Photographs that show you doing things that are important to you. Include snapshots of activities you enjoy doing and things you are good at. Pictures can say a lot about you. They can illustrate your talents, skills, and interests.

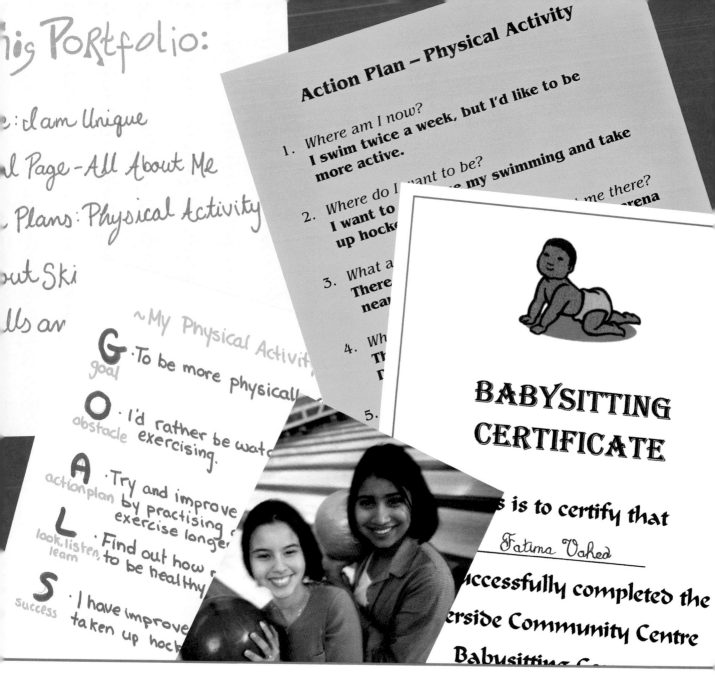

This Portfolio:

Title: I am Unique

Title Page - All About Me

Action Plans: Physical Activity

About Ski

Skills an

~My Physical Activity

G goal · To be more physicall

O obstacle · I'd rather be watc exercising.

A action plan · Try and improve by practising exercise longer

L look, listen, learn · Find out how to be healthy

S success · I have improve taken up hock

Action Plan – Physical Activity

1. Where am I now?
   I swim twice a week, but I'd like to be more active.

2. Where do I want to be?
   I want to my swimming and take up hocke

3. What a
   There near

4. Wh
   **T
   I**

5.

BABYSITTING CERTIFICATE

is is to certify that

Fatima Vahed

ccessfully completed the

rside Community Centre

Babysitting C

- Your goals and action plans. Samples of work you have done up to now to reach a goal.

- Any pages or items about your personal interests.

- Any pages or items about your skills and talents. You can include samples of work, copies of certificates of participation,

awards, merit badges, and anything that makes you proud.

- Information about any other involvement such as volunteer work and teamwork experiences.

- Information about your plans for education and progress.

- Information about careers that interest you.

Using Your Portfolio

What you can get out of using your portfolio depends on what you have put in it. Use your portfolio as an important place to keep valuable information about you. Your portfolio is a **living document,** which means that you can add to it and change it as you change, grow, and have new experiences.

You can use your portfolio to:

- show other people who you are and what you can do

- keep track of how you are learning. When you go through your portfolio, you will be able to review your accomplishments, goals, and plans. When you add to your portfolio, you see what you are learning. Over time, you will see how much you have learned.

- remind yourself of goals that you still want to achieve. Rereading your action plans can jog your memory and keep you on track to meet your goals.

- give you courage to try something new. When you see how much you have learned, improved, and grown, you believe you can succeed at new things.

- keep track of your best work. When you look at what you have done, you can feel proud.

⤷ Over to You

1. Create your own Personal Portfolio. Start by reviewing what goes into a portfolio on pages 136 and 137. Include the information you recorded in the Start Now! activity on page 131. Look throughout this book for the other activities that have portfolio icons 📁 beside them. And add your work from these activities to your portfolio too.

2. When you have completed your portfolio, choose one item or page from it. It could be your favourite thing, something that would interest others, or something you think is most important. Describe what you have chosen. Then explain why you made this choice. What does this item or page say about you? Is it connected to one of your goals? If yes, explain how. If no, explain why not.

Your Thoughts About Future Plans

Your thoughts about the future are a combination of dreams, ideas, and information. The activities you like now can also be part of your "future thinking" because you'll probably continue to enjoy the same ones. People around you can also show you possibilities for your future. Their ideas and attitudes can influence you.

When you think about the future, you might wonder what jobs will be available and what kind of education and training you will need for those jobs. You might consider how much it will cost to learn how to do a job that interests you. You might wonder about the money you can earn if you have that job.

How can you spur on your "future thinking"? Look at your favourite school subjects. Think about how these subjects could relate to activities in your future. Look through your portfolio to remind yourself of your successes, past interests, and all you have learned. Search for new career ideas. Now is the time to think about all the great possibilities for your future.

Why I Am Interested

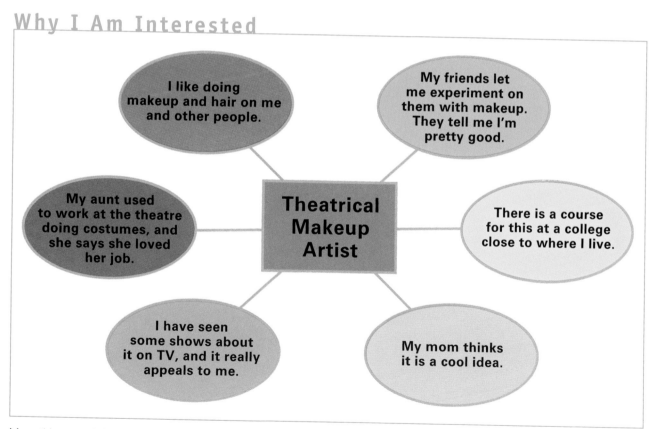

Many things can influence a person's career choice.

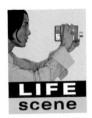

Thoughts About the Future

These days, Brill's favourite activity is sports—any sport, in any weather, with other people or alone. Boarding and soccer are hot right now. It would be great to do stuff like this and get paid for it!

On the flip side, Brill has gone to Saturday art classes at the community centre for three years now and really likes the instructor, who is also an artist. Someday, Brill wants to have a real art show like the one the instructor just had. Having a job as an artist would be great, but is there such a thing? Is it a full-time job?

Brill's mother has worked at the same job for the past 15 years. She says she still loves going to work each day. Brill's father has had about 7 different jobs in the last 15 years. He says he's happy with how it has all worked out. He really likes the job he has now.

Brill's older brothers are twins but very different. Tom is in fourth year at university; Ted is working as an apprentice in a carpentry shop. Both Tom and Ted say they like what they are doing.

Brill does well in school, and one of Brill's teachers has even suggested that Brill apply for a university scholarship. Brill likes the idea of going to university. Training at a technical school or college is also something Brill has thought about.

Brill's favourite school subjects are art, science, phys. ed., and math. Brill wonders how all of these things fit together. Lucky for Brill that the next school project is a career search.

There are many other things to think about. The country's economy is down and unemployment is high, especially in Brill's city. Jobs are difficult to find.

Brill has just finished making a portfolio cover for a school project. Good thing too, because there are many pages waiting to be organized. Brill realizes that it will be helpful to look through the portfolio every so often when thinking about the future. There is a lot to think about.

◀◀ Now You Know

→ Technology creates changes that will affect your future. Education and training must also change to meet new job requirements.

→ There are many things you can do now about the future. You can choose to make plans about future education and career possibilities.

→ You can have goals in many different aspects of your life.

→ Goals should be realistic and meaningful. Action plans help you arrive at long-term goals.

→ One benefit of action plans for long-term goals is that you have time to review your plans and adjust them if necessary.

→ A personal portfolio is one way to organize information about you and what you can do.

⟳ Over to You

1. Choose one career that interests you. Then think about your own answers to the following:

   a) How did you become interested in this type of work?

   b) Why do you think this could be a good job for you?

   c) Why do you like this kind of work?

   d) Write a paragraph that explains why this career is a possible good choice for you.

2. Review the Life Scene on page 140. As you can see, there are many influences on Brill's thoughts about the future. Identify the influences on Brill and suggest some other influences that might affect Brill.

3. Review the diagram on page 139. Then choose a job that interests you. Make a web diagram to show some of the reasons the job you have chosen appeals to you. Think about things in your life that might influence your choice of job.

Answer to Quick Quiz on page 130

Congratulations if you guessed that every idea is real and actually exists. Don't feel bad if you guessed that some of these ideas are fiction. Just a few years ago, some of them were just a dream. Do you have an idea that could become real?

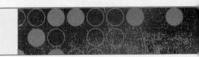

The Immune System

The **immune system** defends your body from illness and infection. Many different kinds of cells, tissues, and organs form the immune system. What you eat and the amount of sleep you get affect how well your immune system works.

1. The **skin** is your body's first line of defence, helping to keep out bacteria and viruses. Blood clots are your body's natural band-aid. They help protect your body by sealing the skin if there is a cut or tear.

2. **Mucous membranes,** such as the ones found in the nose and mouth, trap and destroy bacteria that might otherwise be inhaled.

3. The **tonsils** help to trap and destroy bacteria and viruses.

4. **White blood cells** move around the body and attack infection, bacteria, and viruses. They are formed in the **bone marrow** and must mature before circulating through the bloodstream.

5. The **thymus** helps new white blood cells mature and specialize so that they can protect the body from different invaders.

6. **Lymph nodes** and **lymph vessels,** which are found throughout the body, help keep tissues clean of bacteria and other invaders.

7. The **spleen** helps filter the blood of bacteria, viruses, and old or damaged cells.

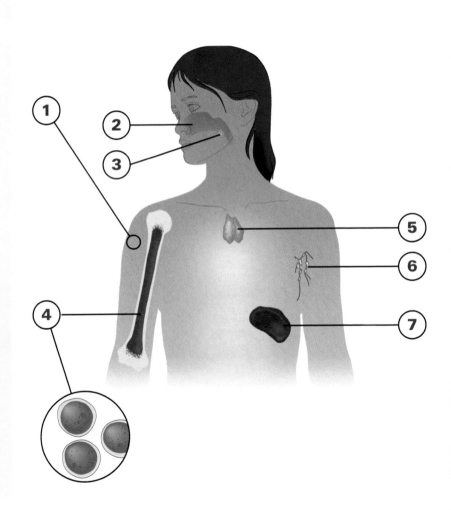

The Respiratory and Circulatory Systems

The **respiratory** and **circulatory systems** work together to absorb oxygen from the air and distribute it throughout the body. Blood is an important part of each system. It carries oxygen and other important nutrients to the body's tissues. Blood also helps remove waste products, such as carbon dioxide, from the body.

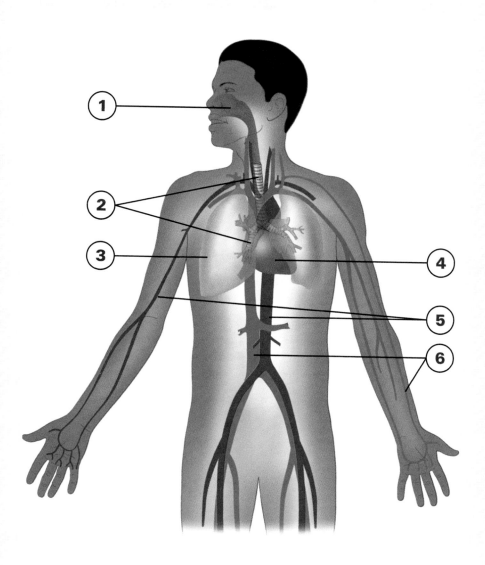

1. Air flows into the body through the **mouth and nose.**

2. The air moves through the **trachea** (windpipe), which branches into two **bronchi,** one for each lung.

3. The **lungs** absorb oxygen from the air and transfer it to the blood. The lungs also remove carbon dioxide when you breathe out.

4. The **heart** is a double pump that moves blood throughout the body. The right side of the heart pumps blood to the lungs. The left side of the heart pumps blood to the rest of the body.

5. **Arteries** take oxygen-rich blood from the heart to other parts of the body. There are also special arteries that feed the heart with oxygen-rich blood.

6. Once oxygen and nutrients have been absorbed from the blood, the blood returns to the heart through **veins.** This blood is then pumped back into the lungs where it absorbs oxygen. The process starts all over again as the oxygen-rich blood is pumped back through the body.

The Digestive System

Digestion is a process that breaks down food into basic parts that can then be absorbed into the bloodstream and used by the body. The body will eliminate whatever it does not need.

1. In the mouth, the **tongue** and **teeth** physically break down food and mix it with the digestive juices in saliva.

2. The food then moves down the tube-like **esophagus** to the stomach.

3. In the **stomach** the food mixes with more digestive juices, which begin to break down the protein in the food.

4. The mixture moves into the **small intestine,** where more digestive juices break down the food into carbohydrates, fat, and protein. These nutrients further break down until they can be absorbed into the bloodstream. Vitamins and minerals are also absorbed into the body through the small intestines.

5. The **liver** makes bile, which helps break down fats.

6. The **pancreas** supplies more digestive juices.

7. Water from the digestive juices and material that cannot be digested move into the **large intestine** and are eliminated from the body.

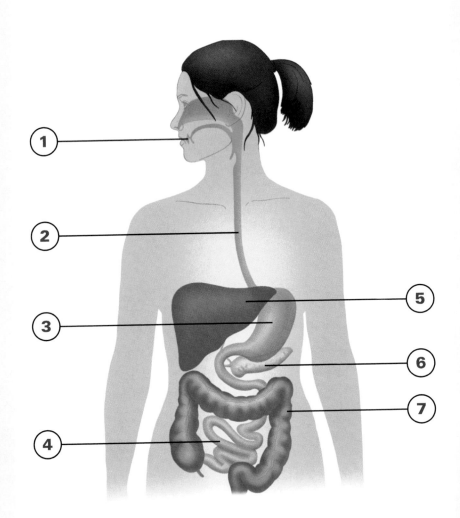

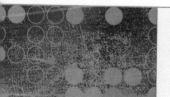

Appendix:
Safety Procedures

Medical Emergencies

A **medical emergency** requires quick action to prevent or limit injury. It is easy to become confused in an emergency. You can help by taking the following steps:

- ❉ Look around to make sure there is no danger to you or the injured person.

- ❉ Shout for help. Get someone else to call the emergency number.

- ❉ If you are alone, then you must call the emergency number yourself.

- ❉ Stay calm.

First Aid

First Aid is the immediate assistance you give an injured person before medical help arrives. Even knowing basic first-aid skills may help you save a life.

Rescue Breathing

An unconscious person may need rescue breathing. Gently tap the person and ask, "Are you OK?" If there is no response and you cannot see, hear, or feel the person breathing, begin rescue breathing.

Rescue Breathing

1. Open the airway by lifting the chin with one hand and tilting the head back with the other hand.

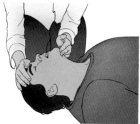

Step 1

2. Gently pinch the nose shut. Maintain an open airway by keeping the chin elevated with your other hand.

3. Seal your mouth over the victim's mouth. Blow in slowly until you see the victim's chest rise.

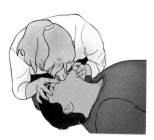

Steps 2 and 3

4. Pause between breaths to allow the air to flow back out.

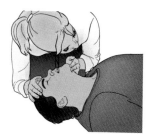

Step 4

5. **Repeat steps 2, 3, and 4** —every five seconds.

6. Continue until help arrives or breathing is restored.

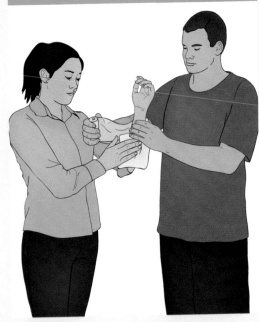

If possible, have the injured person apply pressure to the wound with his or her hand.

Bleeding

1. Apply pressure to the wound with a clean cloth.

2. If the cloth becomes soaked with blood, don't remove it; simply place another cloth on top.

3. Help the person lie down and keep the injured limb raised.

4. If there's something in the wound, such as a piece of glass, don't remove it. Apply pressure around the cut, instead of directly on it.

5. Wrap the cloth with a bandage to hold it in place.

6. For severe bleeding, shout for help or send someone to call an ambulance.

There is little risk that you will catch a disease by touching someone's blood. However, you should wear rubber gloves if possible. If rubber gloves are not available, you can use a plastic bag. If you touch someone's blood, wash your hands with soap and water immediately. It is a good idea to wash your hands right after giving any kind of first aid or assistance to someone.

Burns

1. For minor burns that are red and have blisters, cool the burn with cold running water. Do not use ice.

2. Make sure you see a doctor, even for a minor burn that has become infected.

3. Do not try to clean a severe burn. Cover the burned area with loose bandages in order to keep out the air. Get medical attention immediately.

Poisoning

1. Call for an ambulance immediately if the person is having trouble breathing or is not feeling well.

2. Keep the person warm and provide comfort.

3. If you know what the poison was, make sure you tell the paramedics.

4. Do not touch any container that you think might contain poison.

Choking

If someone starts choking and cannot cough, talk, or breathe, call for help immediately. In the meantime, you can help by performing abdominal thrusts.

Choking

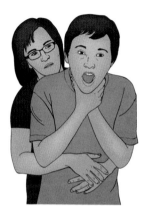

1.

Stand behind the person and put your arms around the person's waist.

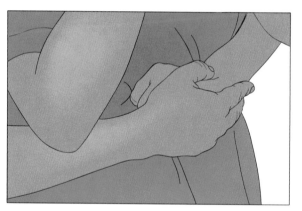

2.

Make a fist with one hand. Place the thumb side of your fist in the middle of the person's abdomen, below the breastbone.

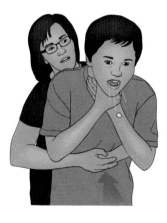

3.

Grasp your fist with the other hand and press into the abdomen with quick upward thrusts. Repeat until the object becomes dislodged.

Glossary

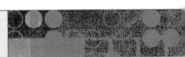

abuse to use improperly

affirmation a positive statement about yourself

all or nothing a pattern of thinking where only your own actions or opinions are acceptable to you

alternative a possibility or option

assertive expressing oneself in a clear, positive, and firm way, without being rude

body image the collection of pictures and thoughts we have in our minds about how our bodies look

bullying pressuring people to do something by making them fearful

circadian rhythms an internal "body clock" that causes people to feel sleepy or awake

coercion the act of forcing someone to do something that he or she doesn't want to do

collaboration working well together to achieve a goal

confidence a belief that you are capable and can be trusted

conform to accept and follow the rules

consequence the result of an action

consumer someone who buys or uses products

feedback response to another person's message

food groups foods with similar nutrients

gang a group of people united by illegal activity and acts of violence

group a collection of people who share something in common

growth spurt a period of sudden and rapid growth

harassment the act of tormenting or bothering someone repeatedly

healthy body image liking who you are

hormone a substance produced by the body that causes some changes or growth

initiation a test someone takes to show loyalty and obedience

intimidate to frighten someone in order to force that person to do something

living document a record of information that you can change by adding new information to it

media different kinds of communication, usually to a large number of people

nutrients substances your body cannot make but does need in order to work properly

overgeneralization thinking that is limited by accepting only one possible result, usually a negative one

peer pressure the strong influence to behave in a manner that is acceptable to others

peers people who have similar interests or abilities

perfectionism a pattern of thinking where a person is not content unless everything is done without any mistakes

personal reflection serious thoughts you have about yourself and your life

personal safety limits your line between what you think is safe and what you think is unsafe

personal standards requirements we set for ourselves

personal values beliefs that are important to you

physical safety protection from danger, physical harm, or injury to the body

portfolio a collection of items organized for a specific purpose

precautions actions a person takes to reduce risk and to be more safe

puberty a stage of development between childhood and adulthood when a person matures

REM sleep the stage of sleep when you dream

resilient having the personal strength to rise above difficult circumstances and adapt to new situations

respect showing consideration for others

risky behaviour taking an action when the consequences of the action are not known

self-talk a private talk that you have with yourself

sleep deprived not getting the amount of sleep each night that is needed to restore a sense of well-being and the feeling of being rested

standard a level of achievement or activity that is required for something to be acceptable

stress tension or pressure that can result in physical and emotional changes

target group a group of consumers that gets special attention because it has money to spend

team a group of people working together toward a common goal

technology the use of new knowledge and discoveries to create new products and processes

thinking pattern the most common way a person thinks about something and explains it

unique being the only one; unlike any other

visualization a picture that you create in your mind

Index

Credits

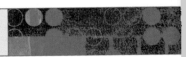

Every effort has been made to trace the ownership of copyright material used in the text. The publisher would be grateful to know of any errors or omissions so that they may be rectified in subsequent editions.

Visual Credits

p. 1 Getty/Stone/Mary Kate Denny. p. 2 Maxx/IndexStock/Patricia Barry Levy. p. 4 Getty/Stone/Stewart Cohen. p. 5 Getty/Photodisc/Jim Arbogast. p. 8 PhotoEdit, Inc./Spencer Grant; PhotoEdit, Inc./Jonathan Nourok. p. 9 PhotoEdit, Inc./Frank Siteman. p. 12 Corbis/Magma/Dex Images, Inc. p. 15 Getty/The Image Bank/Peter Cade. p. 17 Getty/The Image Bank/Todd Pearson. p. 19 Health Canada Web site and Media Photo Gallery, http://www.hc-sc.gc.ca. Reproduced with the permission of the Minister of Public Works and Government Services Canada, 2003; Corbis/Magma/Tom Stewart; Corbis/Magma/Tim Wright. p. 20 Corbis/Magma/Royalty-Free. p. 23 Getty/The Image Bank/Philip Condit II. p. 25 Getty/Taxi/Rob Gage. p. 26 Corbis/Magma/Jose Luis Pelaez, Inc.; Corbis/Magma/Rob Lewine. p. 28 PhotoEdit, Inc./David Young-Wolff. p. 29 PhotoEdit, Inc./Spencer Grant. p. 32 Getty/Stone/Peter Cade. p. 33 Getty/Taxi/Rob Gage. p. 38 Getty/Photodisc/Jim Arbogast. p. 41 PhotoEdit, Inc./David Young-Wolff. p. 42 Corbis/Magma/Tom & Dee Ann McCarthy. p. 49 Getty/Taxi/Rob Gage. p. 50 PhotoEdit, Inc./Myrleen Ferguson Cate. p. 51 PhotoEdit, Inc./Dana White. p. 55 PhotoEdit, Inc./Mary Kate Denny. p. 58 Digital Vision. p. 60 Getty/Taxi/Stephen Simpson. p. 61 OmniPhoto/Esbin/Anderson. p. 62 Getty/Photodisc/Jim Arbogast. p. 64 Corbis/Magma/Richard Hutchings. p. 65 Getty/Photodisc/Jim Arbogast. p. 70 Getty/Photodisc/Jim Arbogast. p. 71 Getty/Photodisc/Michael Matisse; PhotoEdit, Inc./Myrleen Ferguson Cate; PhotoEdit, Inc./Mary Kate Denny. p. 72 Getty/Taxi/Rob Gage. p. 74 PhotoEdit, Inc./David Young-Wolff. p. 76 PhotoEdit, Inc./Mary Kate Denny. p. 77 Getty/Taxi/Rob Gage. p. 78 PhotoEdit, Inc./Tony Freeman. p. 81 Corbis/Magma/Rob Lewine; Getty/Taxi/Ron Chapple. p. 82 Getty/ImageBank/Lars Klove Photo Service. p. 84 Getty/Photodisc/Jim Arbogast. p. 85 PhotoEdit, Inc./Frank Siteman; PhotoEdit, Inc./Spencer Grant. p. 88 Getty/Stone/Joe McBride. p. 90 Corbis/Magma/Dann Tardif. p. 95 SuperStock/Francisco Cruz. p. 96 PhotoEdit, Inc./Michelle D. Bridwell. p. 97 PhotoEdit, Inc./Nancy Sheehan. p. 98 Getty/Photodisc/Jim Arbogast. p. 100 SuperStock/Lisette Le Bon. p. 104 Getty/Photodisc/Jim Arbogast. p. 105 Getty/Photodisc/Jim Arbogast. p. 106 PhotoEdit, Inc./Jonathan Nourok. p. 107 PhotoEdit, Inc./Mary Kate Denny. p. 110 Getty/Photodisc/Jim Arbogast. p. 113 Getty/Photodisc Green/SW Productions. p. 115 Corbis/Magma/Rob Lewine. p. 117 Getty/Taxi/Rob Gage. p. 118 Corbis/Magma/Tom & Dee Ann McCarthy; Getty/Stone/David Young-Wolff. p. 123 Getty/Stone/Lori Adamski Peek. p. 124 PhotoEdit, Inc./Michael Newman; Getty/Stone/David Young-Wolff. p. 125 PhotoEdit, Inc./Myrleen Ferguson; PhotoEdit, Inc./Mary Kate Denny. p. 126 Getty/Photodisc/Jim Arbogast. p. 128 PhotoEdit, Inc./Richard Hutchings. p. 132 PhotoEdit, Inc./Tony Freeman; Will Hart. p. 135 Getty/Stone/Ian Shaw. p. 137 Corbis/Magma/Charles Gupton. p. 140 Getty/Photodisc/Jim Arbogast. Royalty-Free Images: Corbis, Corel, Digital Vision, Getty Images.

Literary Credits

pp. 10–11 Based on the research and application strategies of H. Gardner (his early work with the theory through to his most recent work with Project Zero, in 2001) and some of the work by Johnson and Louis, Dickinson, and Campbell and Campbell. p. 17 *Canada's Physical Activity Guide for Youth,* Health Canada, 2002. Reproduced with the permission of the Minister of Public Works and Government Services Canada, 2003. p. 19 Inspired by the *Handbook for Canada's Physical Activity Guide to Healthy Active Living,* Health Canada, 1998. Adapted and reproduced with permission of the Minister of Public Works and Government Services Canada, 2003. p. 20 Adapted from *Canada's Physical Activity Guide to Healthy Active Living,* Health Canada, 1998. Adapted and reproduced with the permission of the Minister of Public Works and Government Services Canada, 2003. pp. 29, 30, 34 *Canada's Food Guide to Healthy Eating,* Health Canada, 1997. Adapted and reproduced with the permission of the Minister of Public Works and Government Services Canada, 2003. pp. 19, 20, 29, 30, 34 *Health Canada assumes no responsibility for any errors or omissions that may have occurred in the adaptation of its material.* p. 30 Based on information from the Dairy Nutrition Council of Alberta. p.52 Advertising techniques: Based on information from Alberta Milk in collaboration with registered dietitians and nutrition professionals from across the province. pp. 85–86 Concept of resiliency: Based on information from Deirdre Ah Shene, "Resiliency: A Vision of Hope," *Developments* 18, 7 (1999), pp. 2–3. Chapter 6 Information on bullying: Based on information from Barbara Coloroso, *The Bully, The Bullied, and the Bystander* (Toronto: HarperCollins Publishers Ltd., 2002). Chapter 9 Information on gangs from http://www.police.edmonton.ab.ca. pp. 145–147 Based on information from *First Aid: The Vital Link,* The Canadian Red Cross Society, Copyright 2001.